Fighting Diabetes the High Tech Way

A Silicon Valley CEO's quest to save his life with technology

By Gerald C. Hsu and Cindy Janus

Fighting Diabetes the High Tech Way

A Silicon Valley CEO's quest to save his life with technology

By Gerald C. Hsu and Cindy Janus

For additional information, please visit: www.eclairemd.com

ISBN: 978-1-7332583-0-2

A MESSAGE TO THE READER

Neither the publisher, nor the authors are engaged in rendering professional advice or services to the reader. This book is not intended as a substitute for medical advice from a licensed health care practitioner. Any decision involving the treatment of an illness should be made only after consulting a physician. Do not adjust your medication in any way without professional medical advice. The reader should consult his or her medical, health, or other competent professional before adopting any of the suggestions in this book or drawing inferences from it. The authors and publisher specifically disclaim all responsibility for any liability, loss, or risk, personal or otherwise, which is incurred as a consequence, directly or indirectly, of the use and application of any of the contents of this book.

This book is dedicated

to my parents.

Fighting Diabetes the High Tech Way
A Silicon Valley CEO's quest to save his life with technology
Gerald C. Hsu and Cindy Janus

Copyright © 2019

ISBN: 978-1-7332583-0-2

Health

First Edition November 2019
Printed in the United States of America

Website: www.eclairemd.com

Cover and Interior Design: Epicenter Creative

BOOK SUMMARY:

Diagnosed with Type II diabetes at the height of his career as a Silicon Valley CEO, Gerald Hsu spent the next decade relying on prescribed medication to control his condition. Unfortunately, his health continued to deteriorate. Refusing to succumb to a life of insulin injections and dialysis treatments, Gerald took it upon himself to study and learn about chronic diseases and food nutrition. He then combined his newfound knowledge of these areas with his background in mathematics, computer science, physics, engineering, psychology, and business management to create a nonprofit diabetes research organization and a breakthrough diabetes management software system, eclaireMD.

Utilizing the system he developed to identify, assess, treat, and monitor his diabetes, Gerald was able to reverse much of the damage done to his health and reduce the dosages of his medications until he ceased taking them completely. This is a story of one extraordinary man's journey to save his own life and his hope to share his knowledge—and the life-saving, high-tech tools he developed—with the world.

CONTENTS

PROLOGUE 1

CHAPTER 1: Background 4

CHAPTER 2: My Health Episodes... 11

CHAPTER 3: The Wake-up Call.. 25

CHAPTER 4: Year One—Starting My Seven-Year Plan (2010) 32

CHAPTER 5: Year Two—Seeking Medical Professionals for a Long-Term
              Relationship (2011–2012)... 35

CHAPTER 6: Year Three—Dealing With Food Issues (2012–2013) 40

CHAPTER 7: Year Four—Research on Metabolism, the
              Foundation of Health (2014) 45

CHAPTER 8: Year Five—Weight and Post-Meal Glucose (2015)....................... 58

CHAPTER 9: Years Six and Seven —Fasting Glucose (2016–2017) 65

EPILOGUE—Abu Dhabi, United Arab Emirates (December 2017).................... 73

GERRY'S RULES—for Diabetes Management... 79

REFERENCES 81

PROLOGUE

Taipei, Taiwan – June 2001

It started as a slight burning sensation in my chest. The pain steadily increased until it tore me from my sleep. It was the middle of the night, and I was alone in my Taipei apartment during a routine business trip to Asia. I tried to keep rising panic at bay by running through possible causes of the pain. Maybe it was just heartburn? But no—I knew it was something more serious than that.

I had experienced chest pains twice before. The first time was almost twenty years before. I'd been driving to work. The 911 Emergency Dispatcher I called had advised me to pull over and wait for the ambulance. That first wake-up call prompted me to request a job reassignment from Division President to a less stressful staff position under the CEO. My request was denied; my division produced one hundred percent of the company's profits, and I was deemed too valuable to be reassigned. A mere nine months later, the second bout of chest pain came. That alarmed me enough that I finally quit my highly stressful job as a Silicon Valley executive to pursue a dream of running my own company.

Seven years on, I was the CEO of a successful, publicly traded company based in the heart of Silicon Valley, with two thousand employees across nineteen countries. Unfortunately, six of those seven years were spent battling a billion-dollar lawsuit with my former boss and former company, which happened to be the industry-leading competitor. This CEO had a personal vendetta against me; he actively sought to bankrupt my company and put me in jail. Threatening my company, my career, and my life, this lawsuit became the main source of relentless stress for the decade preceding my third attack of chest pain.

That night in Taipei, I realized my condition, whatever it was — was getting worse. I called my personal driver for an emergency ride to the local hospital, which was only two miles away. Thankfully, I had spent the first twenty-one years of my life in Taiwan, so communicating my condition to the doctors in Mandarin Chinese wasn't an issue. However, my mounting fear and dread were more difficult to articulate. I was fifty-four years old and experiencing my third cardiac episode.

They hospitalized me for a week. I couldn't remember the last time I had spent so much time in bed. Until that point, my work had consumed me. My entire life had been meetings, phone calls, problem solving, emergency dealings, and more meetings, with international work trips thrown in here and there. I had become addicted to the adrenaline of it all and was always moving like a high-speed train. This time, I had no choice but to slow down and reflect on my health and life.

Although I was never a smoker or drinker, I had been abusing my body in other ways. Intense stress, lack of sleep, lack of water, and unhealthy high-fat foods (too much food in general) were destroying my body. In my fast-paced Silicon Valley career, I failed to supplement my meals with healthy snacks or drink sufficient amounts of water throughout the day, so when I did finally sit down to eat (usually late at night), I inhaled copious amounts of food like a bear going into hibernation. It was no wonder I developed a forty-six-inch (117-centimeter) waistline on my five-foot-ten-inch (178-centimeter) frame.

Given the distended pot belly that I'd been sporting for over a decade, I had long ago replaced all my belts with suspenders. Some people thought my suspenders were an eccentric CEO's fashion choice. My wife, kids, and I knew the truth: they were purely functional. Wall Street investors nicknamed me "the potato farmer," and I would laugh it off by saying, "It's either these suspenders or imagine a watermelon wearing a belt!" I often used humor to deflect any form of negative attention I received regarding my personal appearance because it was easier to laugh about it than to do something about it.

Looking back on this period, I see that those suspenders were the ultimate embodiment of the Band-Aids I had been using in my life. I was always addressing the symptoms of my poor health rather than the root cause. I'd take antacids for heartburn and prescription medication for diabetes, high blood pressure, high cholesterol, and high triglycerides. When my knees became inflamed from carrying my excess weight, and I could no longer walk-up stairs without pain, I avoided stairs altogether and took the elevator. I even installed an elevator and chair lift in my private residences. I was constantly adjusting my life to make room for my health ailments, telling myself these were the inevitable conditions of getting older. I see now that I was in complete denial about my poor lifestyle choices and habits.

Although I was able to ignore my first two cardiac episodes, the third bout of chest pain in Taiwan—and a fourth that followed a month later—raised red flags on which I couldn't put a Band-Aid. Being the CEO of a company that also happened to be battling a major lawsuit was an all-consuming job, a job I was no longer physically able to do.

As I lay in the hospital bed, questions rushed through my mind. What should I do with the company I had invested all my heart, mind, and body to create? Would I have the opportunity to watch my newborn granddaughter grow into an adult? Although I had spent my entire adult life working toward becoming the CEO of my own, successful company, I knew that, for the sake of my own life, I had to step away. All the long hours I had put in and the sacrifices I had made would have been a waste if I didn't live long enough to enjoy the fruits of my labor. It was a difficult decision. But once the lawsuit was over, I would sell the company.

On my final day in the hospital, I told my family, "I have never given up on a fight in my life. But this time, I received a loud and clear message from God. My life will be near the end if I don't stop. I have to quit fighting for my company and fight for my life instead."

CHAPTER 1

BACKGROUND

I was born in China in 1947. A year later, my family immigrated to Taiwan, a tropical island located about a hundred miles off the southeast coast of mainland China. My father was a Western-trained medical doctor and a Lieutenant Colonel in the Chinese National Air Force. My mother had been a military nurse during World War II and later became a homemaker. I was the third—the middle—child of five. My siblings and I were all raised in Taiwan. I moved to the United States at the age of twenty-one to continue my education, and I've remained ever since as a U.S. Citizen.

For as long as I can remember, I've been a headstrong, determined, and driven individual. My curiosity as a child often caused me to question my parents, asking, "Why?" and "Why not?"—which annoyed my mother greatly. In traditional Chinese culture, children aren't supposed to question their parents or teachers. For my entire life, my mind, which has never been able to relax, has been a blessing and a burden. I'm constantly processing information, questioning things, and figuring out complex problems—and I have a photographic memory, so I retain a lot of information in detail.

This ability to retain and process information has been helpful to me in engineering and business, but it has caused aspects of my everyday life to suffer. For example, I often find myself pondering numbers and graphs throughout the day. Sometimes this happens while I'm driving, which has resulted in a few traffic violations. I've always been an absent-minded driver. This quirk of mine reminds me of the way John Nash was portrayed in the movie A Beautiful Mind. Nash would project the mathematical equations and formulas he was thinking about into his visual sphere; it was as if he was actually seeing the numbers on windows or walls. It's difficult for me to shut my brain off and focus solely on the mundane task of driving when I see numbers and formulas pop into my field of vision.

On the positive side, this ability enabled me to absorb a great deal of material in complex subjects such as mathematics, computer science, mechanical engineering, structural engineering, ocean engineering, finance, and marketing in my undergraduate and graduate studies over a seventeen-year period. Since 2003, I've self-studied abnormal psychology, internal medicine, food science, nutrition, and social psychology, with a focus on behavior.

Coming to America

My early years in the United States were spent in Iowa, Philadelphia, and Boston. While these years helped form my character and develop grit, they were difficult. I endured a lot of hardship in my academic and personal life. My English language skills were inadequate, which nearly caused me to be academically dismissed after my first semester at the University of Iowa. At the time, like many other immigrants, I was poor. In order to support myself through graduate school and to feed and house myself, I worked various physically demanding jobs. I was a dishwasher, waiter, driver, and janitor (I cleaned one thousand toilets in less than nine months). I also faced racial discrimination, once being made to wait eight hours outside a hospital emergency room when I was ill, only to be turned away completely in the end.

My professional career began in 1975 in Connecticut and New York; I worked as an engineer, designing the engine for the Space Shuttle Enterprise and later the building structure and piping systems of nuclear power plants. I worked extremely hard, often staying in the office or a nearby hotel for two to three weeks at a time. During this period, I had a wife and a young son to support, and unfortunately, I rarely saw them. My hard work paid off, however, because by the end of the year, I received a salary increase three times higher than my peers'. I rose quickly within the company, and by my third year I was making twice the average salary of my undergraduate classmates working in the same field.

Eventually, my wife and I decided we could no longer tolerate the long and frigid East Coast winters, so I applied for a position out west. We moved to California in 1976, and I worked for a nuclear power consulting firm in San Francisco. I approached my new position with the same work ethic as before, often sleeping on the floor of my office with a jacket as a blanket and a stack of books as a pillow. I was quickly promoted within the two-thousand-person company, from a low-level technical supervisor to a manager of two separate divisions. Before the age of thirty-five, I became the company's youngest and only non-Caucasian vice president.

Entrepreneurship

Early in my career, a supervisor told me, "Try to be the boss someday. Don't always be a worker." I always kept this piece of advice close to my heart. Like most headstrong and driven individuals, I wanted to prove to myself and the world that I could be a successful entrepreneur. After reaching the VP level at the nuclear power consulting firm, I quickly realized that was as far as I would be able to ascend in that company, because of internal politics. I decided it was time to start my own company.

My first attempt at running my own business had come when I was still living in New York: an engineering consulting firm. However, that business never took off. This time, at age thirty-five, I cofounded a portable personal computer company, which had some moderate success but ultimately went out of business. I didn't have a lot experience in running a business, and, more to the point, we lacked the capital to keep the business afloat during lean times.

Over the next thirteen years, I founded five companies that all eventually failed. In between failures, I went back to work in the corporate world to gain more experience and save capital for my next venture. Finally, in 1994, on my eighth attempt, I hit it big.

Prior to my eighth business venture, I was working as the VP of Sales and the VP of Engineering (a very unusual combination) for the top tech company in a highly specialized industry. After I'd developed a reputation in that company and industry for being a top performer, a venture capital firm sought to recruit me as CEO of a small semiconductor startup. I was being paid quite well at my corporate job, but I still had the passion and dream of running my own successful company, so I accepted the CEO position.

Over the next eight years, I grew this ten-person start-up into a two-thousand-person company that would go on to be publicly traded on NASDAQ and, eventually, would be the top-ranked company in its sector. The success of the company was followed by personal success and recognition. By 2000, Wall Street considered me the most successful Asian-American CEO in the technology sector, and I was the highest paid of the fifteen thousand CEOs in Silicon Valley.

I was proud to have built a company of highly educated and intelligent employees in seventy-two offices throughout nineteen countries. My company employed more than a thousand sales and support personnel and another thousand technical employees with Masters and PhDs from top universities. Since our business dealt in producing the highest-tech components in Silicon Valley, we had to employ the most highly educated engineering and computer science minds in the world.

During the eight years total I served as CEO, I worked an average of one hundred and ten hours per week, usually sixteen to seventeen hours per day. On a typical day I'd wake up at 6 or 7 a.m. and think about work issues during my morning shower and breakfast. Before arriving at the office at 9 a.m., I would be on the phone with my European subsidiaries. From 10 a.m. to 5 p.m., I focused on U.S. operations. From 5 p.m. to 9 p.m., I shifted my focus to operations in Asia. After 9 p.m., I worked with my research and development (R&D) engineering team until midnight or so, then went to bed around midnight or 1 a.m. I would do it all over again starting at 6 a.m.

I worked like a maniac, without taking a vacation or a sick day, for twelve straight years. I distinctly remember taking my daughter on a summer vacation to the northeast right after she graduated from the fifth grade. The next time I took her on vacation was to the northeastern provinces of China after she graduated from university eleven years later. It was clear that I was neglecting my family life; my personal health received even less attention.

Every December I traveled to Japan because it was the only country in which I did business that didn't shut down during Christmas. My favorite time to take a transoceanic flight was on New Year's Day; it was the calmest, most relaxing, and least trafficked travel day. In order to see my family a little more, I'd occasionally bring them with me on business trips, but that didn't mean I spent much time with them.

Stress and Bad Habits

I traveled constantly—on average at least one trip per week due to the vast geographical disbursement of my customers and satellite offices. During this period of my life, I traveled to Japan more than five hundred times. Since I never smoked, drank alcohol, or had any interest in hostess bars, the main form of entertainment with my customers in Asia was going out to eat. I recall one time in Osaka and Kyoto where I had four dinners in one evening (5 p.m., 7 p.m., 9 p.m. and 11 p.m. in a karaoke bar). Overeating during these many lavish meals with my customers and not exercising definitely contributed to poor health and my later development of diabetes.

The stress of working long hours as a CEO was exacerbated tenfold by what was to become the biggest, and most expensive, legal showdown of my professional career. It also happened to be the biggest and most expensive showdown Silicon Valley had ever seen to date.

The CEO of my previous employer, who was also my former boss, called me shortly after I quit and demanded to know where I was working and in what capacity. I responded, "I am the CEO and founder of a newly formed semiconductor company." He was very agitated and told me I absolutely, could not be the CEO of a company in competition with his company, to which I asked, "Why not?" He then yelled over the phone, "Because you are too capable and too dangerous to us!"

I was fed up with him trying to control me during the three years I worked under him and I wasn't about to let him control me after I had left his company, so I shouted back, "This is ridiculous! I came to the U.S. over twenty-five years ago based on the belief in the American principles of freedom and choice. As far as I'm concerned, no one in this world can take this basic right away from me. I'm definitely not going to allow you to take away my choice and rob me of my opportunities. I am going to build a great company and allow our customers to have the freedom to choose between us as well."

Not liking my response, he promised: "I am going to sue you. No, destroy you." I've never been one to back down from a threat or challenge, so I ended the phone call with "Go right ahead!"

Within fifteen months of that phone call, my company became the second most successful Initial Public Offering (IPO) on NASDAQ that year, right after Netscape, a computer services company that pioneered an early web browser. After my many years of hard work and struggle to finally build a successful company of my own, my former employer filed a major lawsuit regarding an intellectual property (IP) dispute. In the complaint, I and five other former employees of the same competitor company were accused of stealing the competitor's code to use in our own company's products.

During the lawsuits, both criminal and civil, that lasted eight years and cost my company approximately $1.4 billion U.S. dollars, I was arrested three times and my name was dragged through the mud by the press. My former boss had lined up five major national television networks and several major newspapers to spread negative news about me and my company. He had also persuaded a local district attorney to do a search and seizure of my company computers in an attempt to uncover evidence and intimidate me.

Having never broken a law in my life, I felt a tremendous amount of stress at being arrested three times for something I didn't do. I felt humiliated at being forced to have my fingerprints and mugshot taken at a detention center, and then being escorted into a jail cell, along with other members of my executive team. We were a group of bespectacled, middle-aged engineers with master's degrees and PhDs from the top universities in the world. We were not a danger to society, yet we were being treated as violent criminals.

As my executive team and I sat in jail that day, I knew, as their leader, I had to maintain my calm in order to boost their morale. I decided to use our time in jail to conduct a strategic business meeting, so there would be no wallowing in self-pity. A prison guard observing us jokingly called me the "ring leader." That day in jail, I swore to myself that I would work harder than I'd ever worked before to earn the billions of dollars we needed to mount our legal defense, protect our reputation and company, and maintain our customers and market share. I knew by keeping the company financially successful, I would win the ultimate war against my former employer.

During those eight long years of criminal and civil legal battles, I learned many lessons regarding the American justice system. The most valuable lesson was that even if a person stands equal before the law and is considered innocent until proven guilty, that person still has a high probability of being found guilty and punished if they lack the financial resources to defend themselves, even if they are innocent. That's why I worked extremely hard every waking minute, and sacrificed my health and well-being during those years, to make good on the vow I made that day in my jail cell. Thankfully, I was found not guilty on all charges, but the damage to my mental and physical health had already been done.

Although the lawsuit is over, it lives on in the form of prominent business and law school case studies. Considered the longest, and one of the most expensive lawsuits in Silicon Valley's history, it coincided with and was a major cause of my deteriorating physical health, which was why I had no choice but to take the drastic measure of selling the company. I had suffered four episodes of chest pain, had developed diabetes, and had a host of other health ailments. Fighting the lawsuit nearly killed me. But I knew I was not ready to die and that I had a lot more to live for and contribute to this world.

Anyone who has spent any time with me knows that I have a hard-driving, never-give-up type-A personality. Having this type of personality has caused me a lot of stress. However, I have never been driven by the desire to acquire power, fame, or money. Instead, my motivation is competitiveness. I've constantly competed against myself because I want today's me to be better than yesterday's me and tomorrow's self to be better than who I am today. It's this drive that eventually led me to shift all my attention and energy from professional pursuits to my personal journey of improving my health and diabetic condition. This is the story of how I did it.

CHAPTER 2

MY HEALTH EPISODES

Until my first bout of chest pain when I was forty-six years old, I never had a health issue that required medication or hospitalization. Admittedly, I was overweight and had occasional insomnia from work-related stress. Nine months after the first episode, the second led me to leave my stressful job as a Silicon Valley executive to run my own company. Despite the stressors of starting and managing a company, I was much happier and more motivated working for myself because I finally felt in control of my own destiny. I was mentally and emotionally where I wanted to be. However, at the time I didn't realize how out of control my physical health was becoming.

At the age of fifty, I felt on top of the world career-wise. I was running my own successful publicly traded company which had just relocated to a beautiful, newly built 90,000-square-foot office on nearly five acres of land by the San Francisco Bay. But my company was also in the middle of a billion-dollar lawsuit. I was working round-the-clock to make sure the company was earning enough to cover expenses.

One day, my body began to shake uncontrollably. I was just sitting at my desk—working through lunch—but my heart was beating very fast. Sweat was gathering on the back of my neck. When I rose from my desk, a wave of dizziness overcame me, and I had to sit back down. Unable to move from my chair, I called for my personal assistant. Her desk was just outside my office. She quickly recognized the symptoms of low blood sugar and brought me a glass of orange juice. Within ten to fifteen minutes, I was no longer shaking.

Still: what the hell had just happened to me? I went to the doctor, who told me I had experienced a classic case of insulin shock. Lack of glucose (an energy source in the form of a simple sugar) and too much insulin (a hormone that regulates glucose) in my blood caused my body to act as though it were starving and to stop functioning. The insulin shock had been precipitated by my skipping breakfast and taking a late lunch. I was later told I was lucky to have experienced only shaking and dizziness; severe cases of insulin shock can lead to seizures, strokes, comas, and even death.

I was confused. I'd skipped many meals before. Never had I experienced anything close to insulin shock. What was going on with my body? My blood was tested over the next several days, and I was diagnosed with severe type 2 diabetes. My doctor used terms like "glucose" and "A1C" to describe my situation. I didn't understand what he was saying. All I wanted to know was how I could get my condition under control with medication so I could get on with my life. I was a busy CEO with a company to run.

My doctor prescribed metformin, the standard and most popular oral diabetes drug of choice. Although I wasn't thrilled about having to take medication every day, I rationalized it as one of the inevitabilities of advancing age. I even considered myself lucky I didn't need to take insulin shots since I hated the sight of needles and blood. Looking back, I see I easily accepted that I was suffering from a chronic disease because my mother, mother-in-law, brother-in-law, and three aunts had diabetes as well. If I had contracted a rare disease, if no one else I knew had suffered from it, I would have felt alone and less positive about the situation. It was okay, I told myself, just a fact of life. Eventually, I came to realize how very wrong I was.

I had spent the first fifty years of my life studying and understanding the complex inner workings of space shuttle engines, nuclear power plants, and integrated circuit chips for hundreds of types of electronics, but I had little idea of how the human body worked. From my general medical checkups, I understood the basic medical terminology of cholesterol, blood pressure, and triglycerides as represented by numbers that were considered either good or bad. Words like metabolism, glucose, and insulin were completely foreign to me. It would turn out that the human body would be the most complex (and amazing) system I'd ever studied.

Understanding Diabetes

The World Health Organization (WHO) defines diabetes as "a chronic, metabolic disease characterized by elevated levels of blood glucose (or blood sugar), which leads over time to serious damage to the heart, blood vessels, eyes, kidneys, and nerves."

As of 2014, over 422 million people worldwide were living with diabetes; in 2015, an estimated 1.6 million deaths were directly caused by diabetes (World Health Organization, 2017). In the United States alone, approximately 29.1 million people (one out of eleven) have diabetes, and one out of four don't know they have it (Centers for Disease Control and Prevention, 2014). Diabetes is a chronic disease that, once contracted, cannot be cured. It can only be managed through diet, exercise, and medication.

The number of people with diabetes has almost quadrupled since 1980, making it one of the leading causes of death in the world. This disease does not discriminate; its prevalence has risen greatly in both developed and developing countries. However, middle- and low-income countries have seen a faster rise than high-income countries, because of rapid urbanization. People who once worked in fields are now sedentary city dwellers with increased consumption of processed food.

Despite how far reaching this disease had become in my lifetime, I was in denial about how serious this condition was and how I, personally, had come to be afflicted by it. To understand why anyone becomes a diabetic, one must first understand how diabetes functions in the body. Basically, diabetes affects your body's ability to produce or use insulin—a hormone produced in the pancreas that helps transport glucose (energy) to your cells. The result is abnormal metabolism of carbohydrates and elevated levels of glucose in the blood and urine.

Insulin and glucose work like old-fashioned steam locomotives to power the human body. These trains need to burn a fuel, such as coal, to speed up, climb hills, and stop at stations. The faster the speed and the longer the distance the train travels, the more coal it needs. The railroad fireman's job is to shovel coal into the engine's firebox and make sure the train is burning the correct amount of fuel for its level of activity. I think of my body as a train that travels and climbs every day. The food I consume is turned into a fuel, known as glucose, for my body to use immediately or store for later use. Insulin is the railroad fireman who shovels the glucose into the cells (firebox) for use as fuel.

Now imagine a train with carts full of coal, but without a fireman feeding coal into the engine. Without the fireman helping to convert the coal into fuel, the train can't run. This is what happens when the body doesn't produce enough, or any, insulin. The body doesn't run. This is the very definition of type 1 diabetes (previously known as insulin-dependent, juvenile, or childhood-onset diabetes). Type 1 diabetes (T1D) occurs when the body's immune system attacks the pancreas to the point that it can no longer produce insulin. Unfortunately, T1D cannot be prevented, but it can be properly managed once diagnosed.

In type 2 diabetes (T2D), the situation is different. The body becomes insulin resistant, which is typical of type 2 diabetes (previously called non-insulin-dependent, or adult-onset diabetes). T2D is, around the world, what the majority of people with diabetes have and is generally a result of lifestyle choices. That fortunately means T2D in many cases can be prevented, delayed, or managed. Genetics do play a role in T2D; however, poor lifestyle choices speed up the rate and severity in which an individual develops the disease.

While not all people with T2D are overweight, the majority are. That included me, when I was first diagnosed. Excess body fat contributes to insulin resistance in the body, which is why obesity has been linked to the development of T2D. Continuing with the train analogy: a fireman can't do his job if the engine room gets too hot or crowded (i.e., insulin resistant). An engine room may become too hot because the engine hasn't been properly maintained or the train has been carrying too heavy a load. If you've been feeding your body more junk food than health food, have not been exercising regularly, and are carrying excess weight (especially around the belly area), then your cells, or engine, may become overheated and insulin resistant.

The third type of diabetes is gestational diabetes, which afflicts some pregnant women. This is the only type of diabetes that can be reversed (after the birth of the child), although, in some women, gestational diabetes turns into T2D after the child is born. Having gestational diabetes also increases a woman's risk of developing T2D later on in life. Also, when gestational diabetes is poorly managed during pregnancy, it increases the health risks for the child during pregnancy and delivery, as well as the risk of the child developing diabetes.

The general signs and symptoms of diabetes are increased thirst; frequent urination; extreme hunger; unexplained weight loss or fatigue; blurred vision; dry, itchy skin; slow-healing sores; increased infections (e.g., gums, skin, and vaginal infections); and numbness or tingling in the feet. Diabetics may have one or more of these symptoms before they are diagnosed, or they may have no signs at all. Before I was diagnosed, I exhibited many of these symptoms but had falsely attributed them to work-related stress. The power of denial is strong, especially if you're unaware of what you should be looking for.

Each type of diabetes has characteristics that are similar to and different from those of the other types. This applies to causes, symptoms, and treatment. Since I have no personal experience with T1D or gestational diabetes, this memoir will focus on my experiences with T2D.

Why Me?

After I came to understand what diabetes was and how it worked inside my body, my next question was "why me?" Why do some people get diabetes and others don't? Although there is currently no definitive answer to that question, diabetes researchers have discovered that certain factors increase the risk. These include family history, race, age, weight, inactivity, high blood pressure, and abnormal cholesterol and triglyceride levels. Other risk factors, specifically for women, include having had gestational diabetes and polycystic ovary syndrome (a hormonal disorder that affects the ovaries).

The first red flag or early warning sign for the possible development of diabetes later in life is family history. Your risk of diabetes increases if a parent or sibling has diabetes. Although we can't control what is passed down from our parents, we can take steps in our personal health to prevent or delay the onset of T2D. This is the first piece of knowledge I wish I'd had before my diagnosis.

I am a combination of genetics from both my parents. But I had always viewed my father as the blue-print for the physical male I would become. He had always been tall and lean, with excellent posture, and I had grown up with a similarly lean build. After he quit smoking in the late 1970s, he was the picture of perfect health. He slept ten hours every night, consumed home-cooked meals that were primarily vegetable-based, took walks after each meal, drank alcohol sparingly, and kept his mind sharp through reading, reciting poetry, and playing mahjong and Chinese chess. My four siblings and I thought he was going to live to one hundred because he had the healthiest habits of us all.

My mother, on the other hand, had always been plump. She had a penchant for sweets and enjoyed richer, meat-based dishes. In the years leading up to, during, and following World War II, she had been deprived of many luxuries, so when she moved to the United states in the late 1970s, she indulged her sweet tooth. By the time she reached her mid-fifties, she was diagnosed with T2D. All I knew about diabetes back then was that it happened to some people and not others, and that medication was prescribed to manage it. It never occurred to me that the condition was likely to pass down to me or my children someday.

Despite my father's healthy lifestyle, he passed away at the age of eighty-eight, two weeks after experiencing his first stroke. The stroke left him brain-dead, but his body remained healthy and functioning while on life-support. Five years after his death, my mother passed at age eighty-one from complications of her diabetes. In the last months of her life, doctors discovered that cancer had spread throughout her organs. My parents had lived with me during the last two decades of their lives, so I personally witnessed their challenges with aging as well as my mother's struggle with diabetes. I never questioned why my father had a stroke or how diabetes killed my mother. They both lived into their eighties, which I considered to be a long life, so I reasoned that strokes, diabetes, heart attacks, cancer, and the like were all inevitable, if one lived long enough.

It's true that the risk of developing diabetes and other medical conditions increase with age (Yale School of Medicine, 2010). However, other factors contribute more heavily to the risk. In the United States, ethnic minorities are two to four times more likely to die from diabetes than are non-Hispanic whites. Basically, if you are African American, Latin American, Native American/Alaska Native, Pacific Islander, or Asian American (like me), you have an increased risk of developing diabetes (U.S. Department of Health and Human Services Office of Minority Health, 2016). The findings are similar in Canada (Diabetes Statistics in Canada, 2017). Researchers are still trying to determine why this is so, but part of the current hypothesis is that many of these groups are afflicted with higher obesity rates and experience socioeconomic factors that attribute to obesity.

The correlation with obesity leads me to what I believe are the two biggest risk factors: weight and inactivity. These two factors often cause or contribute to the other risk factors of high blood pressure, high cholesterol, and high triglycerides. When it comes to diabetes, these symptoms are all related, and they compound each other.

My father, who had never been overweight a day in his life, did not have diabetes. His father, my grandfather, had been a farmer, so daily physical activity was a part of my father's lifestyle while growing up. My mother, whose weight stayed on the higher side most of her life, developed diabetes at age fifty-six. She came from a wealthy family, so she had access to richer foods from an early age. Also, as a female growing up in China during the early twentieth century, she was not encouraged to engage in physical activity outside of domestic housework. I believe these lifestyle factors that they experienced while growing up contributed to my parents' adult weights and activity levels.

Growing up in Taiwan, I was always thin and physically active. My family was not wealthy, so we never owned a car and had to walk everywhere. Only when I was in college did I start riding a bicycle. Our meals consisted mainly of white rice, tofu, fish, and vegetables. Eating meat was rare, and we never had the luxury of red meat. Once I moved to the United States at age twenty-one, red meat was readily available everywhere and at affordable prices, so I began to indulge. Steaks, hamburgers, hot dogs, meat loaf, sausage, roast beef, corned beef, ribs, and the like became my staples. (I had stopped eating poultry at a young age after my mother butchered my pet chicken for dinner).

In Taiwan, I had never exercised for the sake of exercising. Physical activity was simply built into my daily routine. Once I moved to the United States, I owned and drove a car for the first time, and that became my main mode of transportation. After finishing graduate school, I had chosen a career in engineering and computers, which, for the most part, involved sedentary tasks most of the day. From my early twenties to early forties, my weight remained within a normal range, as defined by the Body Mass Index (BMI). But at the age of forty-four, I began to notice significant weight gain, especially in the abdominal area. My arms and legs were still relatively skinny, but I was definitely growing a pot belly. By the time I was forty-seven years old, I had traded in my belts for suspenders.

My diagnosis of severe T2D at the age of fifty probably meant I had been an undiagnosed prediabetic in the years leading up to it. Diabetes is known as the "silent killer." It creeps up on you, at first without symptoms. Often, outward physical symptoms don't show up until you've already had diabetes for a while. This is why it's so important to get regular checkups and blood tests. I had not been getting regular doctor checkups so I didn't know my A1C (average blood glucose level over the past ninety days) levels.

The A1C blood test is used to screen for and diagnose prediabetes and diabetes. It measures how much glucose is attached to your hemoglobin (a protein in red blood cells that carries oxygen). If you have a 5 percent A1C level, that means 5 percent of your hemoglobin proteins have glucose attached. A normal A1C range is considered 5.7 percent or less. An A1C range for prediabetes is 5.7 percent to 6.4 percent. An A1C range for diabetes is 6.5 percent or above. In terms of A1C levels, I like to think of glucose as a potentially clingy sweetheart. Glucose is great in small, steady doses because he or she is sweet and full of energy, but too much clinginess causes damage to a relationship. In fact, 5.7 percent and above of this glucose clinginess causes damage to the body.

Starting Medication

When I was first diagnosed as a severe type 2 diabetic, my A1C was around 8 percent. My blood glucose levels were out of control, so the doctor prescribed an oral medication called metformin. Metformin is supposed to help reduce the amount of glucose produced and released by the liver, and to increase insulin sensitivity. Diligently, I took metformin every day—and still, my A1C bounced between 7 percent and 9 percent. The doctor kept increasing my dosage. Eventually, he added a second medication, pioglitazone (brand name Actoplus). And then he added a third medication, sitagliptin (brand name Januvia).

Now taking heavy dosages of three medications, I never questioned if there were other ways to manage my condition. My doctor had given me the perfunctory "eat-better-and-exercise-more" speech, but there was a lack of a detailed plan and true call to action. I'm not blaming my doctor; I could have pushed for more guidance. After all, it was my life, and if I didn't take charge of it, no one else would. However, my focus and priorities at the time were so completely on my company and the lawsuit that I had put on blinders about my disease, hoping medication would make it go away. Denial can be the most self-destructive force there is.

By the age of fifty-three, I had been on three medications for four years and I was getting worse. While I was on a business trip to Taiwan, my body finally had enough. My third episode of chest pain came in the middle of the night. After being hospitalized for a week, I did some soul searching. If I wanted to continue to live, I needed to drastically change my lifestyle, and I knew that meant selling the company I had worked so hard to build. I loved what I did; I wanted to continue leading the company. But my body would not be able to handle it.

After being released from the hospital in Taiwan, I made arrangements to return to California. However, I became concerned that the fourteen-hour flight from Taipei to San Francisco be too much for my heart. I decided to take a nine-hour flight to Honolulu instead, and to rest there for a few weeks. During my time in Hawaii, I experienced another bout of chest pain and landed back in the emergency room. Finally, my heart condition stabilized, and I flew back to California. From the time I left Taipei to when I arrived in San Francisco, an entire month had passed.

I felt I had no time to waste. The morning after I arrived, I called a special board of directors meeting and announced I would resign from the position of the president and CEO, although I would remain as the chairman and chief strategic officer. In these positions, I would handle only strategic matters (such as a merger), not day-to-day operations. After resigning, I began preparing to sell the company and planning to move to Asia. Ten months later, the company was acquired by a competitor, and I was able to exit the fast-paced, Silicon Valley lifestyle for good. I regard this as one of the smartest decisions I've made.

And yet I was still operating like a high-speed machine. My mind and body had become so accustomed to running on adrenaline that at times I could still taste the extreme bitterness in my mouth—an outpouring of adrenaline accompanied by low blood sugar can cause a metallic or bitter taste in the mouth. Every time I experienced this bitter taste, I felt as if I was literally being poisoned by stress.

Just because I had sold the company and moved to Asia, it didn't mean I actually knew how to relax or slow down. I had spent my entire life working and hadn't developed any outside hobbies or love of leisure activities (other than eating at restaurants). It was never my intent to retire and travel or start playing golf. What I enjoyed doing—and the only thing I knew how to do—was to work. Without any real reflection, I launched two new nonprofit projects overseas. I still lacked an off button.

The first project, called Software Robotics, used software to develop programs automatically. I spent a total of nine years (from 2002 to 2010) completing the development of this technology and its prototypes. Also, as a result of feeling mentally and emotionally traumatized by my lawsuit, I began reading about abnormal psychology. In the years 2002–2003, I pored through sixty-four textbooks and five hundred clinical papers in this area, and my eyes were opened to other people's traumas, particularly that of women and children.

Thus, my second project, launched in 2003, eventually led to the creation of four psychotherapy centers in Taiwan to help abused women and traumatized children. I started by touring different institutions for physically abused women and children in Japan, since I was living in Asia at the time, and Japan had the most developed trauma infrastructure I was aware of in the region. Taiwan, I realized, had few equivalent institutions, I decided to start my own nonprofit psychotherapy centers. I'm proud to say these centers helped over one hundred women and children. That number may seem low compared to numbers in the United States, but consider that in many Asian countries, like Taiwan, there is a heavy stigma in seeking help in these matters or admitting to a problem in the first place. If only one woman or child had been helped through my endeavors, I would have considered it a success.

My version of retirement was to work on things I enjoyed doing, such as innovation, research and development, and helping people. Instead of fighting legal battles and dealing with the endless pressure of Wall Street, I now had the time and means to pursue my passion projects. However, although I had changed my line of work, I hadn't altered my lifestyle enough to truly address my deteriorating health. I felt like a car that speeding recklessly down a road towards a brick wall. Although I was no longer going full speed, I was still cruising on the same road and in the same direction. I needed to change directions before I hit the wall.

Living in Asia

I believed that eating more Asian food would improve my diet. After all, I had grown up in Taiwan and obesity had never been an issue there. In general, people in Asian countries are slimmer than those who live in the United States. However, I now know the problem wasn't just about food. Most people in Asia do not own cars. They have to walk, bike, or take public transport, which makes a major contribution to health. Even in Japan, where I know many people who own cars, driving is expensive because of highway tolls and parking fees. Many of my acquaintances there walk and take public transport most of the time.

So living in Asia didn't automatically make me like most people there. I was now a spoiled American. Although I enjoyed walking, I didn't enjoy doing it in the humidity, heat, high winds, or rain. I had personal drivers, and I utilized them whenever it suited me. Although I'd purchased a treadmill for my office, I rarely used it. I was having a lot of knee pain because of being overweight, so I told myself I would exercise more after I lost weight.

Meanwhile, the bad habits and excuses were keeping me from losing weight. True, portion sizes in Asian restaurants were smaller than in the

United States—so I would simply order three or four portions. I still had my American-sized appetite. Also, as I later learned, Asian food is not healthier for diabetics. I'll address this in more detail later in the book.

With my weight and glucose levels still out of control, I needed to take drastic measures. My first course of action was to hire a dietician. She came to my office and began advising me on the things I should and shouldn't be eating. I rebelled. Because she appeared to be overweight, I thought: who is she to tell me what to do? I disregarded her advice and went back to looking for another quick fix (i.e., medication).

One day, my doctor in Taiwan told me about hospital-prepared diabetic-friendly meals for purchase. I jumped at the opportunity. My driver would pick up my pre-packaged lunch and dinners from the hospital and deliver them to my wife and me every day. The meals consisted of an animal-based protein (a quarter of my plate), a half-cup of white rice (a quarter of my plate), and some type of cooked vegetable (half of my plate). Salt and oil were used minimally. I found the meals decent at first, although lacking in flavor. With my portions under control, I finally began dropping weight. My glucose levels improved. I was ecstatic and thought all my troubles were solved!

During the first month of eating those hospital meals, I cheated only occasionally, usually when I had to take a visitor to dinner or when I traveled on business. But after the first month, the meals felt tedious, and I began snacking between meals and late at night. Before I knew it, I had gained back all the weight I had lost. By the end of the third month, I stopped ordering the hospital meals and went back to my old ways.

Back in the Emergency Room

At age fifty-seven, just two years after selling my company, I was back in the emergency room after experiencing my fifth episode of chest pain. My driver had rushed me to the Taiwan University Hospital, which was the top medical facility on the island. The doctors gave me MRIs and other tests, finally concluding that I would need open-heart surgery within two days. They wanted to place a stent (a tubular support structure) to widen my arteries so more blood could pass through. This news scared the hell out of me. I asked them to hold off on surgery until I could speak with my primary physician in California.

My U.S. doctor preferred I not have open-heart surgery in Taiwan. After verifying I was healthy enough to return to California, he encouraged me to fly back immediately with my test results from Taiwan. After interviewing three heart surgeons in the Bay Area, I selected an intelligent and skillful surgeon in his early forties, who worked with a good cardiology team at the San Ramon Regional Hospital. This surgeon wanted to do a coronary angiogram first, which is a special X-ray test to find out if, where, and how much my coronary arteries were blocked or narrowed. I went under general anesthesia, and a long, thin tube called a catheter was inserted into an artery in my groin area and threaded up to my heart. A special fluid went through the catheter so that my arteries would show up on the X-ray and my doctor could see where the blockages were.

The entire procedure took less than forty-five minutes. After I woke up, the surgeon said, "There's good news and bad news. Which one do you want to hear first?" I told him I wanted to hear the good news first, so he said, "You are fifty-seven years old, but your heart is as young as the heart of a forty-year-old man."

That was fantastic news! Then I asked him what the bad news was.

He replied, "The bad news is that you have an abnormal heart. A normal heart has three major arteries, one in the front, one on the side, and one on the back. The artery on the back of your heart never developed. However, God created the human body to do amazing things. Your body sensed that you didn't have a back artery, so the two existing arteries automatically developed numerous branches to cover the entire back portion of your heart." As he told me this, he drew a representation of my heart and arteries on a piece of paper.

Lying in my recovery bed, I thought about all the people in my life who had commented on my special heart. They meant the way I put my heart and soul into my work, building companies and helping people. Now I realized I literally had a special heart. I was strangely proud of that fact. To this day, I've kept that drawing my doctor made of my heart as a reminder that being abnormal isn't always a bad thing and that the human body has a miraculous capacity to heal itself.

The surgeon went on to explain that my missing back artery was probably the reason why the doctors in Taiwan had misdiagnosed me. After digesting the fact that I'd almost had unnecessary open-heart surgery, I asked my doctor why I'd been having all these bouts of chest pain. He replied, "Based on your business background and your lifestyle, your heart has suffered a tremendous amount of stress. It's time for you to wake up and change your lifestyle completely. Otherwise, you may not be so lucky next time."

Once again I was being told by a doctor to change my lifestyle. I still had no idea what that truly meant. I thought selling my company, moving to Asia, buying a treadmill, hiring a dietician, and eating hospital meals was changing my lifestyle. I've since learned that a real lifestyle change didn't just mean changing my line of work and my address, and buying new things. I needed to change my way of thinking, and my relationship to diet and exercise. In other words, changing my lifestyle meant changing the priorities in my life and, thereafter, changing all of the related tasks, activities, and habits associated with my new set of priorities.

CHAPTER 3
THE WAKE-UP CALL

I'm a very stubborn person with a type-A personality. I like to do things on my own terms and am always seeking the fastest possible route to my goal. While these traits may have helped me become a successful CEO, they also slowed my progress towards a healthier lifestyle. Used to seeking quick fixes, I was looking for that magic bullet that would cure me. I was too impatient to stick with any course of action I felt wasn't yielding immediate results. On top of that, I was battling a lifetime of bad habits, like overeating, not regularly exercising, and drinking very little water.

I continued this internal battle without making any real changes to my lifestyle until the age of sixty-three. That year, during a routine checkup, I learned that my A1C had reached an all-time high of 10 percent. My urine albumin test or albumin/creatinine ratio (ACR), which is used to screen for kidney damage, had reached 116 mg/mmol. That was four times higher than the maximum allowed value: in a normal person, the ACR should be less than 30 mg/mmol. I was sixty-three years old and on my way to complete kidney failure.

Improperly managed diabetes, it turned out, affects your entire body, and that includes your most important internal organs. The kidneys are a pair of bean-shaped, fist-sized organs located in the back on each side of the spine. They filter waste products from the blood and are involved with regulating blood pressure, electrolyte balance, and red blood cell production. In the United States, about one out of every four adults with diabetes have kidney disease (National Institute of Diabetes and Digestive and Kidney Diseases, 2016). Diabetes is the number-one cause of kidney failure because, over time, high blood glucose damages the blood vessels in the kidneys. Also, many diabetics develop high blood pressure, which also damages the blood vessels in the kidneys. When your kidneys are no longer working properly, or stop functioning all together, dialysis treatments are needed.

Dialysis replaces kidney function by removing waste products and excess fluid from the body. The machines are expensive and fairly large; to get treatment, most people must go to dialysis centers or hospitals at least three times a week. Patients lie on a recliner with two needles inserted near the wrist. One needle draws the blood into the machine to clean it, and the cleaned blood returns through the other needle. This process takes approximately four hours. Four hours, three times a week, plus the time it takes to commute to and from the center—dialysis is a part-time job that doesn't pay.

My doctor said I would most likely need to undergo dialysis treatment within the next three years. He also advised me to go on insulin shots right away to control my blood glucose levels. This was the moment I finally woke up. Maybe I didn't have the best understanding of my diabetic condition, but I knew what dialysis was, and I was horrified.

My brother-in-law, also named Gerry, had been diagnosed with T2D at the age of twenty-six and, twenty years later, because of the severity of his condition, had passed away. At the time of his diagnosis, he was a priest, serving amongst the Taiwanese aborigines in the mountainous regions of Taiwan. Because of the nature of his vocation and the location where he served, he did not seek out medical knowledge or medications to manage his disease until after he left the priesthood in his early thirties. In the relatively short time I knew him, I witnessed him go through numerous operations on his eyes, heart, and feet. In the last five years of his life, he was on dialysis. He was confined to a wheel chair the last few years of his life and was only forty-six years old when he passed.

As I witnessed his painful journey, I also noticed the heavy burden that his deteriorating health placed on my sister and their young children. During Gerry's last days, I remember sitting next to his bed at the hospital and holding his hand while he asked me to take care of his two young daughters, aged ten and eight. With tears in my eyes, I promised him I would look after my sister and their daughters. I knew I was capable of taking care of them financially, but at that moment, I had no idea how I could fulfill the role of a missing father.

When my doctor said I would eventually need dialysis, my mind flashed to images of Gerry on his death bed. It finally dawned on me that having diabetes was more than just my own health care issue; it involved all my loved ones who cared about me and depended on me. Although my children were grown, as well as my nieces, whom I had assisted financially while they were growing up, I knew I still needed to be there for them, as well as for my wife. I had two grandchildren by my son whom I wanted to watch grow up. I wanted to walk my daughter down the aisle at her wedding. I had so much to live for, and when I pictured myself getting insulin shots four times a day and going three times a week for dialysis treatments, I was terrified I would miss those special moments while also bringing down their quality of life.

I was sixty-three years old. My doctor had just told me I would most likely be dead in five years if I didn't make serious changes. Nevertheless, when he urged me to start insulin injections that day, I refused. First of all, I had serious misgivings about turning my body into a laboratory by pumping chemical compounds into it for years on end. Second, I questioned whether the current medical community truly understood all the potential side effects of daily insulin injections. And finally, I couldn't stand the thought of using needles on myself every day. To this day, I still hate the sight of needles and blood.

As I drove home after my appointment, all I could think about was how both my parents had lived into their eighties and my doctor was telling me I wouldn't reach seventy. I felt as though I were experiencing all five stages of grief at the same time: denial, anger, bargaining, depression, and acceptance. By the time I reached home, I decided to do what I always did best, which was to fight. I felt the only option for me at this point was to fight my prognosis. In order to fight, I needed more knowledge and a plan.

Once and for all, I decided to dedicate my focus and energy to reversing the deterioration of my health. I approached this undertaking as if I was building my last company. I was going to be the successful CEO of my own body, and I was going to use all my knowledge, resources, and stubbornness to save my own life.

Since I'd had some short-term weight-loss success with packaged diabetic meals in Taiwan, I set about searching online for a similar service in the United States. I typed in "ready-made food for diabetics" and found a company in Atlanta, Georgia, that prepared pre-cooked, frozen meals for diabetic patients and would ship them anywhere in the United States. I decided to purchase a one-month supply of meals that I could carry with me to Las Vegas, where I was headed next to purchase a house.

Viva Las Vegas

About a year before, a friend had introduced me to a nice, large suburb in metropolitan Las Vegas, where many other retirees lived. After decades of visiting the Las Vegas Strip for business conferences and trade shows, I was delightfully surprised to discover such a large, residential community of professionals and retirees living nearby. While walking in my friend's neighborhood, I was overcome with a feeling of peace. Observing the blue, cloudless skies and temperate weather, I felt this was a place I could live.

When I lived in Silicon Valley, a feeling of stress would overcome me as I drove from my house to work in daily traffic. If I went to a restaurant to unwind, I would hear people around me talking about business and technology, constant reminders of work. I felt constantly enclosed by people and things that caused stress. There was no stress associated with living in Las Vegas.

It was now August 2010, about two years after the financial crisis. Real estate in Las Vegas was still down by 50 percent. It was the perfect time to buy a house. Armed with a big box of frozen diabetic meals, I flew there and rented a suite with a kitchen at a business hotel near the Strip. I spent the next three days house hunting, and when I found the house I wanted, I made an all-cash offer on the spot with a request to include all the existing furniture in the deal. The seller accepted my offer, and I arranged for a cleaning company to clean the house the following day. On my fifth day in Las Vegas, I moved into the house. I felt I had no time to lose and wanted to move in right away so I could focus solely on my health.

During my first month in my new home, I concluded that the first priority was to rid myself of all work-related stress. Although I had sold my publicly traded company in 2002, I was currently managing two nonprofit or not-for-profit organizations with seven hundred employees across four countries. Even though these not-for-profit entities did not need nearly as much attention as my previous software company, I still encountered numerous financial and management issues which caused me stress.

This decision was difficult enough in the case of my not-for-profit technology project. I had spent the past eight years developing innovative technology in the field of software robotics, and we were on the verge of commercializing it. Now, without the physical capacity to see this technology through product refinement and commercialization, I had no choice but to shut down operations. It was the right thing to do, but I struggled with this decision for about a month.

However, the decision to close down the nonprofit psychotherapy centers I had set up in Taiwan hurt my heart the most. I had received an immense amount of satisfaction from helping abused women and traumatized children, and I wanted to do more.

With a very sad heart, I called my management team to let them know my decision. I followed up the phone call with a message to all my employees via a simple, but clear email. "I am facing life or death at this moment," I wrote, "and therefore, I cannot continue what I intended to do. Effective now, I will shut down all of my operations." I've always been a very honest and direct communicator, and it would have been disingenuous of me to write a long and flowery message. Instead, I chose to get right to the point because I felt my employees deserved to know the simple truth; their boss would die if he didn't step away now.

In my experience, when a business shuts down so suddenly, it can face all kinds of trouble and litigation from disgruntled employees. I didn't encounter any trouble at all. Every one of my employees realized that I was facing a life-or-death situation, and they respected my decision. Within a week, I was able to shut down all business activities across all four countries. I'm forever grateful to these former employees for their understanding and support.

It was now my third month in Las Vegas. While I sat in my study and stared out the window at the desert and the beautiful skyline of Las Vegas, I thought about the following questions: How can I reverse my current physical condition? What kind of plan should I have? Who can help me? After a lot of soul searching, I came to the conclusion that no doctor had been or would be able to apply traditional methods of treatment to cure me. There was no miracle drug.

I had been a diabetic for over ten years, I had reached the near-maximum dosage of my diabetes medications, and my symptoms were only getting worse. A small cut on my toe turned into an infection that required antibiotics and three months to heal. Diabetics typically have poor circulation, especially in the lower limbs, causing wounds in those regions to heal very slowly. This is very dangerous for severe diabetics because their wounds are slower to close, and the rate of infection is higher. Infections of this type can lead to the amputation of toes, feet, or legs.

I was horrified by the thought of losing my feet or legs to this disease. Amputation is a treatment of symptoms, designed to avert death; I was more interested in preventive medicine. Scouring the internet for information on reversing diabetes, I came across alternative herbal treatments used by Eastern or Chinese medicine. However, I chose not to pursue that path because of the lack of scientific support. Eventually, I concluded that if I could not cure my diabetes, I could at least keep it from getting worse. At this point, I simply wanted to increase the quantity and quality of my remaining years.

I've always been the type of person who takes it upon himself to learn what I need to know. Early in my career, when I was hired to manage a structural engineering team that was designing a nuclear power plant, I took soil engineering courses at the local university and immediately began applying what I learned in class to my workplace. When I was promoted to the Division Manager of Financial Systems, with no background in business or finance, I took night MBA courses at a university down the street from my office. My approach to learning and applying knowledge to my immediate situation has served me well in my career, and I believed I could do that with my diabetes as well.

If I had been younger, I might have decided to attend medical school, but I didn't have enough time for that. Anyway, I didn't need a medical degree to save myself. In fact, I believed I could regain my health through simple determination, focus, knowledge, and persistence. Those were the ingredients that allowed me to succeed in business. Confident I could transfer my approach to business to my health, I decided I was the only person who could help me. I had to depend on myself to save my own life.

CHAPTER 4:
YEAR ONE
Starting My Seven-year Plan (2010)

My fundamental approach to saving my life was to research human biomedical behaviors related to diabetes. Examples of behaviors related to diabetes include eating (food quantity, quality, and time of consumption), drinking water, sleeping, exercising, experiencing stress, smoking, consuming alcohol, and more. These behaviors are all aspects of a patient's lifestyle. After deciding what to research, I began putting together a seven-year work plan that would run from 2010 to 2017. I chose seven years because that's the typical amount of time required to complete a Ph.D. program in engineering at a prominent university. In the beginning, I chose to focus the project on diabetes and five interrelated chronic conditions: hypertension, hyperlipidemia, heart disease, stroke, and obesity.

Anyone can read about these chronic conditions on the internet or in a textbook; I wanted to delve deeper into the science, so I decided to study internal medicine on my own. Since I had determined I was too old to go to medical school and my current physical health demanded I make progress quickly, I decided on a short cut. I would read medical textbooks on my own and hire medical professionals as consultants. They could help fill in the gaps in my knowledge and help guide my research.

When I was the CEO of a high-tech company, I hired and surrounded myself with the best and brightest minds in electrical engineering and computer science. These elite-class professionals and I worked together to create and commercialize the most sophisticated high-tech tools available in the world. The technology we created was utilized by millions of individual consumers, companies, banks, and the military. I was excited at the prospect of now surrounding myself with the most highly educated medical professionals to help find the answers to my problems. I was still an engineer at heart, and true engineers seek practical solutions to real-world problems. I was not interested in sitting around debating the theoretical reasons why diabetes exists and how to manage it. I wanted concrete, scientific proof that if I applied A, B, and C factors, I could control my diabetes through X, Y, and Z outcomes.

Finding high-quality medical professionals in the United States who would work with me turned out to be difficult. Most top American medical professionals are already consumed with their own practices or research, or both, and do not have time to be consultants. I was an unknown entity with no medical background to speak of; people were naturally skeptical of working with me. In fact, at the start of my seven-year plan, I met a few medical doctors who laughed in my face: how could I conduct a personal diabetes research study without possessing a medical degree?

Since I had successfully sourced talent from Asia in my previous nonprofit ventures, I decided to seek medical consultants in China. The Chinese medical system is set up differently from the U.S. one, and I reasoned that I would be able to find more medical consultants willing to help. Also, the costs of hiring these individuals would be lower. What I didn't realize at the time was that sourcing medical experts in China was very different from sourcing engineering skills and talent in China.

I spent the entire year of 2011 traveling back and forth between Las Vegas and China, working with eighty-two local medical professionals there. During that time, I was working with my software engineers to develop tools on the iPhone so that I could begin inputting my personal health data (i.e., daily glucose levels and weight). During the software development process, one of the doctors I was working with suggested developing an automatic diagnosis system for lung disease. Without thinking it through, I took him up on his suggestion—and got sidetracked. I spent the next year learning how to diagnose diseases that were not specifically diabetes-related, and my medical team completed an automatic diagnosis system for lung disease related to bronchitis and pneumonia. I was heading in the wrong direction.

How could I have strayed so far?

The medical field was new to me. When there's so much you don't know, many things may at first appear interesting and relevant. After all, all parts of the human body, from blood and organs to bones and nerves, work together and affect each other. I halted all my efforts with my medical team in China, and returned to my home to the United States to regroup.

My year of working on my medical project in China made me realize that the practice, research, and ethics of Western medicine were still developing there. China had reopened its doors to the Western world only about forty years ago, and it was a Communist country, which meant the free flow of information and innovation was still limited.

I had enjoyed living in Las Vegas. During my time there, I had met other retirees. For the first time in my life, I had attempted to develop some hobbies outside of work. I'd even joined a choir. However, old habits die hard. Las Vegas wasn't the best place for me to focus on my research studies, and what I needed most was to work. Most of the retirees around my age suffered from chronic illnesses like diabetes, with varying severity of symptoms. I found it depressing to be around others who thought socializing meant complaining about their bodies falling apart. I still felt twenty years old at heart, and I sincerely believed the next stage of my life would be even more exciting than the last. Whenever I talked about my research and my belief that I would reverse my diabetes, the other retirees would look at me with strange expressions and dismiss my seemingly grandiose ideas. I had spent my entire life as a can-do spirit and big thinker. It felt incredibly frustrating to be around people who couldn't see my vision. Even though most of us had the same disease, diabetes, I still felt alone because I was the only one who really wanted to do something about it. To me, diabetes was not a death sentence, but a challenge to live my life better.

So, after leaving China, I returned home to California.

CHAPTER 5

YEAR TWO

Seeking Medical Professionals for a
Long-Term Relationship (2011–2012)

Sitting in my dining room on Thanksgiving Day, I stared out at the calm San Francisco Bay through the window. Looking into the distance always gives me a sense of peace and clarity. On that day, I felt I was literally looking ahead of me, to where I needed to go and what I needed to do. I noticed that I was gazing directly at the city of Palo Alto across the water. Palo Alto is the home of the Stanford University School of Medicine, one of the top five U.S. medical schools for research (U.S. News & World Report, 2017). It was in that moment that the idea of establishing my research center near Stanford University came to me.

I quickly called over three of my previous work acquaintances, including Dennis Heller, my right-hand man from my Silicon Valley CEO days. The four of us gathered around my dining room table to discuss the idea of forming a company to help people manage diabetes. Despite our lack of background and knowledge in medicine, we were knowledgeable enough to know this new venture should address two important issues associated with diabetes: body weight and glucose.

After settling on this new focus, we discussed where the business should be physically located. Dennis advised me not to spend money on renting a big, fancy building. Instead, I should take the traditional Silicon Valley approach of bootstrapping the operation from our own garages (in my case, a home office suite). Despite the tremendous financial success Dennis and I enjoyed from my old Silicon Valley semiconductor company, we had both become more fiscally conservative, though for different reasons.

In my case, after I sold my company in 2002, I had invested millions of dollars into a software robotics project. Although the project gave me a great deal of personal satisfaction from a technical standpoint, it had no financial return. In Dennis's case, he had joined a struggling startup company and internalized the importance of creating a thrifty start-up culture. To this day, I appreciate the cost-savings advice he gave me that day, which I'm sure saved me from wasting millions of dollars.

This thrifty approach helped transform me from an engineer/businessman into a scientist. Instead of hiring medical experts to work on this project, I personally did almost 90 percent of the work. This work included studying various subjects, reading research papers, developing concepts, designing the system, collecting and analyzing data, deriving equations, testing and debugging software, generating graphics, and writing a medical paper. The only task I didn't personally do was software programming because my time would be better spent in other areas. I spent about 18,000 hours over seven years on the diabetes project. If I had charged for my labor at a discount rate of $100 per hour, this project would have cost nearly $2 million.

A year earlier, when I'd launched the company, I had wanted to hire top U.S. medical professionals to guide me in my research. Instead, I sourced less expensive medical professionals from China, which didn't yield the results I had hoped. I realized if I wanted to make strides in my research, I had to associate with professionals who held power and authority within the Western medical system—and this thought was what led me to Stanford. The medical school at Stanford University had been established twenty-seven years before the actual university was established in 1885. To me, this meant, Stanford Medicine was the nexus of Western medicine and research on the U.S. West Coast.

I knew that Stanford-trained or -employed medical professionals might not be interested in working for or with me, but that didn't mean I couldn't build personal connections with them as friends. It's my belief that when you are in the prime of your life and building your career, you should have friends who are lawyers and accountants. These professionals can help grow your career. But, as you get older and have more physical ailments, it's best to have friends who are doctors. Now that I'm seventy years old, I have more friends who are doctors than I've had at any other time in my life.

Since I didn't personally know anyone at Stanford Medicine, I decided to begin networking with doctors in two ways. The first approach was to move closer to Stanford University and switch to a primary care physician who worked at Stanford Medical Center. Even if my personal diabetes research never went anywhere, at least my personal health would be overseen by the best. My second approach was to place an advertisement on Craigslist. My ad read, "Medical doctor wanted for a nonprofit organization to conduct research on diabetes and other chronic diseases."

I had only recently learned about Craigslist (I had been living in Asia when Craigslist became a household name in the United States), and I didn't know what type of individuals I would attract. I was pleasantly surprised when I received six responses from doctors living in Silicon Valley, Los Angeles, Cincinnati, and Toronto. Of these, half were experienced clinical physicians who were curious about my intentions, and the other half were newly graduated interns who needed a part-time job to pay off student loans. Three of the respondents had received their professional training from prestigious institutions: Stanford University; the University of California, San Francisco (UCSF); and the University of California, Los Angeles (UCLA).

The Birth of eclaireMD

Having just turned sixty-five, I was ready to get back to researching and understanding diabetes, hypertension, hyperlipidemia, heart disease, stroke, and obesity. I pored through online public information from only the most reputable and reliable sources, including Harvard Medical School, Johns Hopkins School of Medicine, Stanford School of Medicine, UCSF School of Medicine, Mayo Clinic, National Institutes of Health (NIH), Centers for Disease Control and Prevention (CDC), World Health Organization (WHO), and American Diabetes Association. I didn't trust any sources that didn't come from the most reputable medical schools, hospitals, federal government agencies, or United Nations–related organizations.

As I was studying the six chronic conditions I'd chosen, I simultaneously began developing a smart phone app to collect my personal health data, including daily weight, post-meal glucose, blood pressure, and so forth. I developed this app, which I named eclaireMD, primarily for my personal use, but I always thought other diabetics could eventually use it. Therefore, I wanted to create a simple platform for users to access needed information, collect their health data, analyze that data, and utilize the resulting feedback to control their diabetes.

I had been working with an outside consultant on the design of the app's user interface design when he asked what I planned to name it. We discussed a few options before finally deciding on eclaireMD. When he found out my previous software robotics project had been named eclair (after the classic French pastry), he suggested I simply add an "MD" behind that name and apply it to my new app. I always liked the word eclair because, to me, it represented things that were small but packed a big punch. Éclair pastries are small but very tasty and flavorful. Software is also small in size, but has the ability to affect you in a big way. Then we decided to add an "e" at the end of éclair, because, in French, with an "e" on the end, the word means "enlightened." Hence, eclaireMD, a small app on your phone with the power to enlighten and change your life.

Since I wanted eclaireMD to operate on both Apple iPhones and Android devices, I needed a software team. So I flew to China and invited the three best software engineers who had worked on my previous software robotics project to my hotel lobby. I brought them up to speed on my current health condition and what I had been working on since disbanding the robotics project. Since the layoff, none of these engineers had found steady work they were passionate about, and they were excited to be a part of my new project. I hired them on the spot, and we began work on eclaireMD immediately. In the process, I taught them how to shift gears from working on software robotics to my new medical analysis project.

My work on software robotics hadn't gone to waste after all. I applied a lot of the original design concepts from that project to the eclaireMD medical software, and I like to think I transported the old eclair software robotics spirit into my new eclaireMD venture.

While setting up the infrastructure of my new nonprofit diabetes research organization and software management system, I continued reading numerous medical textbooks and research papers on the six chronic diseases I was focusing on. The more I read and researched, the more I formulated my strategy on how to attack and manage my diabetes the high-tech way.

CHAPTER 6
YEAR THREE
Dealing With Food Issues (2012–2013)

I quickly learned that food is the most prominent factor in controlling one's glucose levels. Out-of-control glucose is what causes damage to the body. Since I lacked knowledge of food and nutrition, I decided to purchase numerous books on the subject and seek out Ph.D.s in food science on Craigslist.

One of the best books I read about food science was *Sugar Salt Fat: How the Food Giants Hooked Us* by Michael Moss. The book discussed how sugar, salt, and fat are the most commonly used additives in the American diet and how, in large quantities, they cause great damage to human health. It is no surprise that many restaurants, especially fast food chains, use very high amounts of sugar, salt, and fat in their food because these ingredients taste good and are highly addictive.

According to Daniel E. Lieberman, chair of the Harvard Department of Human Evolutionary Biology, many of the current health problems we face in this country arose from an evolutionary mismatch: humans evolved over many centuries to live on a hunter-gatherer diet that consisted of fruits, vegetables, nuts, seeds, plant roots, and the occasional lean meat and fish. Large quantities of sugar, salt, and fat were hard to come. But because sugar and fat are very efficient sources of energy, humans became evolutionarily wired to prefer those tastes. Since farming was invented, humans have been able to stay in one place and eventually develop technologies that provide copious amounts of food that are not found in nature and that contain highly addictive additives. Human biological evolution is very slow. Our bodies have not caught up with our new diet, which is much heavier in sugar, salt, and fat. This is why obesity and diabetes rates are growing all over the world.

While educating myself on food science, I realized I needed a nutrition guide to help me understand what I was eating on a daily basis. For example, if I ate a medium-sized banana, I wanted to know how many calories and grams of carbohydrates, protein, fat, sugar, and sodium it contained. While many nutrition guides were available via the internet and other apps, I wanted to access all this information on my own app. It would be easier and faster to look up the nutrition of a banana and add it to my food diary on the same app, instead of looking it up elsewhere and having to input it. I decided to develop a food and nutrition database for eclaireMD.

First, I purchased the food composition database from the U.S. Department of Agriculture (USDA). Second, my team went online and collected up-to-date menus from approximately five hundred U.S. chain restaurants. On average, each chain restaurant had about two hundred menu items with sixteen important nutritional ingredients listed for each. Finally, I integrated the chain restaurant data with the USDA database to form the initial food database for eclaireMD. Eventually, the eclaireMD database expanded to include close to six million data points relating to food and nutrition.

While I as proud of the fact the app had so much food and nutrition data available, I realized the data needed to be organized so that users could quickly find what they were looking for. I went back to Beijing, China, and hired two hundred college students, on summer break, to clean up the data. My three software engineers developed an eclaireMD search engine to enable and facilitate information accessibility. However, there was still a gap in the database.

Making Better Food Choices Through eclaireMD

I believe it's common knowledge that cooking at home is generally healthier than eating at restaurants. Restaurants rely on heavy doses of sugar, salt, and fat in order to make meals taste good so that patrons will return. While occasional meals at restaurants are fine, the unfortunate reality is that the percentage of Americans eating outside the home has risen steadily since 1970, reaching its highest level of 43.1 percent in 2012, the year I developed eclaireMD (United States Department of Agriculture Economic Research Service, 2017). In fact, as of 2016, retail sales at U.S. eating and drinking establishments have outrun those of grocery stores (United States Census Bureau, 2016).

With so many Americans were eating their meals in both chain and independently owned restaurants, I knew the key to helping users make better food choices was to have a comprehensive food database. Gathering food and nutrition data on chain restaurants was relatively easy, as they normally publish this information on their websites. However, independently owned restaurants presented a challenge because of the wide variety of chefs, recipes, and ingredients. These restaurants typically didn't publish (and weren't even aware of) their nutrition data. It took me a few months to think through this dilemma, but my engineer mind finally came to a practical (and simple) solution.

Most restaurant owners, chefs, and cooks (including home cooks) are not food nutrition experts. If you were to ask the average restaurant cook how many calories from carbohydrates, fat, and protein were in a specific meal, I doubt they would know. Generally speaking, they are in the business of making food taste good, not making it healthy. Therefore, diabetics who cook at home or eat at restaurants with no published nutrition information are responsible for educating themselves on basic nutrition components and portion sizes.

One day, while I was taking my daily walk and thinking through this dilemma, I came to a couple of conclusions. First, for diabetics, keeping track of the amount of carbohydrates and sugar consumed is the most important factor in keeping glucose levels in check. Realizing portion control was the heart of the matter, I suddenly recalled a conversation I had with a Taiwanese dietician fourteen years earlier, when I'd first been diagnosed as diabetic. The dietician had advised me to eat only one bowl of rice and half an apple (if the apple was larger than my fist) at each meal.

As I walked, I looked down at my hand and balled it into a fist. I realized that the dietician had been trying to educate me on portion control using a low-tech measurement tool—my hand. Thinking of the famous American Express credit card advertising slogan, "Don't leave home without it," I realized that no matter how forgetful people can be, they never leave home without their hands. This simple, yet practical technique for estimating food portions was the answer to my dilemma!

I quickly made my way home and began an internet search for the average American height and the ratio between palm size to height. Based on these measurements, I developed a method of utilizing the palm, fist, finger, and thumb to measure food portions. My team and I went to the supermarket and purchased a variety of raw foods, including beef, pork, chicken, fish, shrimp, and various vegetables and grains. We then cut and measured the food into specific sizes corresponding to an adult palm, fist, finger, and thumb. After weighing the food on a scale, we took photos, and recorded the information for the eclaireMD food database. During the next two months, my kitchen became our food science laboratory.

I stored this food in my freezer so I could continue to experiment on myself. Every day, I consumed meals from my freezer so that I could match my post-meal glucose levels with the raw or cooked food I ate. At the same time, I became obsessed with building my food database and wanted as many photos of a variety of whole, raw vegetables as possible. I went into numerous supermarkets to take photos of vegetables and was even stopped by a store clerk once because he thought I was a spy from a competing supermarket.

Second, as I continued to develop my food estimation system for eclaireMD based on photos and hand measurements, I realized some users would not be able to accurately identify all carbohydrates. Generally, when you ask someone to name a carbohydrate, that person will say "bread" or "pasta." This is correct; however, carbohydrates exist in many other forms outside of flour-based products. For example, before I started my food nutrition studies, I had no idea that fruits and vegetables contained carbohydrates. I had been under the impression that all fruits and vegetables were healthy and could be consumed without limit. While fruits and vegetables are healthy, they cannot be consumed without limit by diabetics, especially potatoes, corn, and bananas.

It was through this lengthy process of trial and error that I came up with the method of having app users estimate the amount of carbohydrates and sugar in each meal based on the size of their palm or fist. Rather than focusing on protein or calories, they would simply identify the carbohydrates and sugar in their meals and measure them against their own hand for portion control.

In addition to portion size, the type of carbohydrate matters as well. A carbohydrate in the form of an unprocessed vegetable has a different effect on your body than a processed-flour-based carbohydrate. Eventually, I completed my food and nutrition database project, but I still wondered how to help users easily and accurately select vegetables and their portion sizes in order to predict their post-meal glucose.

After much trial and error, I developed a color-based selection table of vegetables which can accurately predict post-meal glucose values. On that table, different foods are assigned different values based on the amount of carbohydrates they possess. This way, users can make conscious choices about what foods to eat based on how those foods will affect their glucose levels.

For example, using one fist or palm size of carbohydrates in the form of bread, potatoes, or pasta is assigned a value of 100 percent, which is equivalent to 20 grams, or 17 mg/dL, glucose points. Green vegetables are assigned a value of 40 percent. Red vegetables are assigned a value of 60 percent. Yellow vegetables are assigned a value of 80 percent. Finally, purple or dark-colored vegetables are assigned a value of 100 percent. In order for diabetics to manage their condition, it is very important for them to understand the values assigned to each food and to consume larger quantities of low-percentage carbohydrates (e.g., vegetables) than high-percentage carbohydrates (e.g., bread) or meats in their meals.

CHAPTER 7

YEAR FOUR

Research on Metabolism, the Foundation of Health (2014)

Nearly four years into my seven-year plan, I finally felt ready to begin my own research on diabetes and lifestyle management. It took me almost an entire year to conduct this part of the research and development because it involved a lot of mathematical modeling and software development. Although I had an undergraduate degree in applied mathematics and multiple engineering degrees that involved heavy mathematics training, most of my professional career as a businessman only required the arithmetic level of a fourth grader. Basic addition, subtraction, multiplication, and division had sufficed. For example, I managed all my businesses using the following four simple formulas:

(1)   Revenue − Cost = Profit

(2)   Profit − Taxes = Net Profit

(3)   Net Profit/Number of Shares = Earnings Per Share (EPS)

(4)   EPS x Price − Earnings Ratio (P/E Ratio) = Total Market Price or Capital (Stock) Value

Having spent the past seven years conducting research and working on a solution to my diabetes problem, I've come to realize that while my head is good at business and my spirit loves literature, art, history, and philosophy, I have always remained a scientist and engineer at heart, always seeking truth through data-driven evidence and practical solutions to real-life problems.

Metabolism

I spent the entire fourth year researching overall health in relation to the chronic diseases I was focusing on. Since metabolism plays a fundamental role in these diseases, I wanted to develop a mathematical model that simulated the human metabolism. To start, I tried to find a good working definition of metabolism—and failed. The Merriam-Webster Dictionary defines metabolism as "the chemical changes in living cells by which energy is provided for vital processes and activities and new material is assimilated." In other words, it's the rate at which your body expends energy or burns calories. That definition does make sense, but it wasn't adequate to my purpose. I needed to be able to quantify metabolism since I was developing a mathematical model for it.

I decided to run my dilemma by a doctor I had recently met and befriended in California. She began her explanation of metabolism by using the word "enzyme." I asked her to explain in plain English. She then characterized metabolism as "energy level," so I asked her to define what a person's energy level was and how it could be quantified in order to manage it. Unfortunately, she wasn't able to answer my questions; in fact, I realized, many of the doctors I spoke with didn't truly understand what metabolism was or how to measure it. Metabolism as "energy level" or health condition (which I expand on later) is ultimately accurate. A lack of depth in the understanding of it frustrated me, however.

My point isn't to blame the doctors, but to shed light on how the current model of medicine is centered around diagnosing and treating disease (people who are already sick), rather than preventing disease in the first place.

Conventional medicine—also known as Western, or mainstream, medicine—operates on a disease-based model. The U.S. medical education system trains doctors to address disease by treating symptoms through medication, radiation, and surgery. Most doctors I have encountered do not have a deep knowledge or understanding of metabolism and food nutrition, and their scientifically established correlation with chronic diseases, such as diabetes. In fact, quite a few of the doctors I met with were overweight and suffered from poor health due to stress, lack of sleep, and lack of exercise.

Diabetics like me have difficulty getting healthy using the current model of medical care because doctors are constantly pushing medication as the first line of defense. It should be the last. Doctors' diet and exercise recommendations can be vague, and they usually take a backseat to medication—even though lifestyle changes should predominate. When a patient begins treatment with medication, the body eventually adjusts to the initial dosage and then it needs higher dosages to maintain the desired results. Often, medications have undesirable side effects, which may result in additional medications being prescribed to manage these side effects. It's a vicious cycle. In my opinion, being pumped full of expensive medications with no end date is not the definition of healthy living.

Glucose Levels

My app, in addition to measuring metabolism, needed to be able to measure and predict glucose levels. The standard way for diabetics to manage their condition is to measure their blood glucose levels via finger-prick blood tests when they first wake up in the morning (fasting glucose), before meals, and two hours after the start of a meal (post-meal, or postprandial, glucose). The American Diabetes Association recommends that diabetics monitor and log their blood glucose levels on a daily basis so that health care providers have a good picture of their patients' response to care plans (diet, exercise, medication, etc.).

At this point, you may be wondering why I developed technology to predict glucose levels when diabetics can use daily finger-prick blood tests to determine their exact glucose levels. The first reason relates to my reason for refusing my doctor's advice to go on daily insulin injections. After having been on three types of diabetic medication in heavy dosages for over fifteen years and still not having my glucose levels under control, I realized I needed to create a treatment that would work for my particular body. Since diet and exercise are key to managing diabetes, I wanted to develop a tool that could tell me exactly what A and B inputs (food and exercise) I needed in order to get the X and Y outputs (glucose levels and weight) I wanted. I came up with my prediction tools was so that I could manage my diabetes without medication or insulin injections.

The second reason I developed this technology was so that I could eat a varied diet without having to worry that if I ate the incorrect foods or portions my glucose would spike. I think many diabetics end up eating the same foods over and over again because they know those meals won't adversely affect their blood glucose. It's easier and safer than experimenting. While some are fine with this type of diet, I am the kind of person who becomes bored without variety. Armed with my app, I'm able to go to any restaurant, input my meal into eclaireMD prediction tools, and know exactly how it will affect my blood glucose before I take my first bite. This, in turn, helps me make wise choices while dining out or eating foods that aren't part of my normal diet. In other words, my glucose prediction tool is a navigation guide for diabetics. A diabetic eating at a new restaurant without my prediction tools would know only after the fact whether the meal had spiked their glucose or not. That's like playing Russian roulette with your meals. I'm not willing to take that chance with my health.

The final reason I developed this alternative blood glucose measuring method was that I passionately hate the sight of needles and blood. Back when I was in high school in Taiwan, I got selected through the Taiwanese national examination to study either medicine or mathematics at university. Although a medical degree would have been more prestigious and lucrative than a mathematics degree, I chose math. It didn't involve needles or blood. Almost half a century later, when my doctor told me to monitor my daily glucose levels using the finger-prick method, I tried to find an alternative method so that I could measure glucose without drawing blood but had no success. My glucose prediction models enabled me to avoid drawing blood every day.

Please note that, in order to conduct my research, I still had to perform finger-prick testing four times a day, on a daily basis. Over the past five years, I've tested my blood glucose this way over eight thousand times. My index, middle, ring, and baby finger pads have been pierced more than a thousand times each. It's one of the small sacrifices I've made in the name of scientific research.

Another benefit of my prediction tools is that they can reduce the costs associated with treating diabetes. By using my tools, many diabetics may be able to cut back on expensive medications and equipment (i.e. finger-prick lancets and test strips) as I did.

As I developed these tools, I realized that eclaireMD would be most useful to diabetics living in developing countries because they are more likely to be constrained by limits on financial resources and access to medications. My prediction tools potentially could be very beneficial to them. This became one of the main motivations behind the further development of my prediction models.

The great thing about software technology is that it often brings down the cost and waste associated with hardware products. For example, e-readers have driven down the costs of reading and the physical production of books. My hope is that my technology can drive down the costs associated with diabetes by helping people manage glucose, weight, and overall health.

There are currently quite a few for-profit companies developing glucose testing and data-collecting devices for diabetics. In my personal opinion, the current model of profit-driven products for diabetics is not solving the problem of diabetes in a fundamental way, nor does it really benefit diabetics in the long run. Instead of profiting off the misery of diabetics, society should be focusing on creating revolutionary ideas and methods to fundamentally control the cause and the growing epidemic of diabetes through the model of preventive medicine.

The Governing Equation

Everyone's metabolic rate varies according to several factors, including age, gender, genetics, and the proportion of muscle to fat in the body. Since eclaireMD's first purpose was to help me improve my own health, it made sense to develop the mathematical models on my own metabolic rate first, and then generalize them to a larger population. In other words, I needed to develop a "governing equation" based on my metabolism. A governing equation is a mathematical model that describes how the values of the unknown or dependent variables will change.

When I first explained what a governing equation was to my son-in-law, he said, "Oh, you mean it's like a recipe?" I thought that was a great way to explain it. Let's say I want to make a chocolate cake, but I don't have a recipe. I eventually figure out through trial and error that a chocolate cake requires flour, baking powder, sugar, eggs, milk, and cocoa. However, in order to perfect my recipe, I need to continue to adjust the measurements of each ingredient until I make the perfect chocolate cake. In this analogy, the governing equation is the recipe I have derived in order to move forward with determining my perfect outcome for my health. By continuously tweaking my inputs and monitoring the resulting outputs, I can figure out the right governing equation.

In this case, my post-meal glucose values were the resulting outputs. Initially, if I ate a meal of steak (4 ounces) and mashed potatoes (one half cup) for dinner, I would not know what my post-meal glucose level would be without a blood test. Once I figured out the math behind my body's glucose behavior, I could simply enter my meal of steak and potatoes into my app and it would use the built-in governing equation to tell me what my glucose levels would be. I needed to start somewhere in order to make the key technology of my app—the prediction model— work, and my body would be the first test subject.

Experimenting With Variables

To do any kind of mathematical modeling, you need a set of numbers to work with. I chose to collect my own glucose data as the basis for the mathematical calculations I would make. My first experiment involved eating the same meal every day, at the same time of day, for thirty days straight. I went to the Denny's chain restaurant near my house and ordered their Salisbury steak with mushroom sauce, with a side of steamed vegetables, garlic bread with butter, and soup. I varied the amount I ate each day to see how portion size affected my post-meal glucose levels, but I always ate the same meal, and I monitored my daily glucose levels with a traditional blood glucose meter (finger-prick method).

Because my prediction model takes me as a baseline, other users can't just pick up my app and immediately begin using it to accurately predict their own post-meal glucose levels. Everyone's metabolic rate is different, which means our glucose behaviors are different. My wife and I can have the same Salisbury steak meal, measure our post-meal glucose at the same exact time, and end up with completely different glucose levels. Therefore, a user must collect and enter his or her own glucose data (taken from traditional blood glucose meters) for the first ninety days so that the app can self-learn the new biomedical conditions of the user and readjust the mathematics accordingly. Users do not have to eat the same meals that I did. They simply need to enter the meals they do eat and the corresponding glucose measurements after each meal. My app uses artificial intelligence to learn about users through the values they input, and then it adjusts predictions accordingly.

This first experiment at Denny's was successful in helping me determine my glucose behavior, but that didn't mean I understood the mathematics behind metabolism. I spent the entirety of 2014 trying to understand, define, and develop a mathematical model that could simulate human metabolism.

Early in the process, I came up with the idea of modeling human metabolism using the finite element method (FEM), which is a numerical method for solving engineering problems. FEM breaks down a large problem into smaller parts. Once you figure out the simple equations of the smaller parts, you can put all the simple equations together to form a model of the whole problem. I had learned many concepts of nonlinear structural engineering during my graduate studies at MIT, including FEM, and I felt I could apply some of those concepts to figuring out the human body.

Metabolism was the large problem that needed to be broken down into smaller parts. Basically, human metabolism was one giant equation, and I was trying to figure out this equation through reverse engineering, by measuring and examining the things that affect and result from the metabolic process (i.e., inputs and outputs). I came up with the governing equation of metabolism based on the quantitative relationships between six inputs (food, exercise, stress, sleep, water, and daily routine regularity) and four outputs (weight, glucose, blood pressure, and lipid levels, which include cholesterol and triglycerides). To discover the quantitative relationship among these ten categories, I relied on advanced mathematics.

One of the equations I wrote out by hand took up eleven pages. When I showed this handwritten equation to two engineer friends from my MIT days, they got very excited about the idea of applying engineering concepts and solutions to a biomedical problem. I, too, was very excited about applying engineering methods I had learned over four decades ago in a completely new scenario that would lead to saving my own life.

After spending the majority of my career as a businessman, I'd thought the only benefit from my early engineering training was the ability to manage engineers in a business setting. In fact, my engineering studies laid the foundation for my approach to solving real-world problems in many areas beyond the nuclear power structures, space shuttle engines, semiconductor electronics, and various software projects I'd worked on. I've also applied everything I had learned in mathematics, physics, computer science, business, and psychology. The longer I live, the more I see that if we pay attention and use our imagination and creativity, we can apply what we have already learned in our lives to help ourselves and others.

The Metabolism Index (MI) and General Health Status Unit (GHSU)

By the end of the fourth year, I had successfully completed my metabolism model. It included two newly self-defined indices, which I termed the Metabolism Index (MI) and the General Health Status Unit (GHSU). The MI is a snapshot of a person's total health condition based on six input and four output categories of the human body's health data. As a reminder: the six health inputs were exercise, water intake, sleep, stress, food and meals, and daily routine regularity. The four health outputs were body weight, blood sugar, blood pressure, and lipid levels. It was only later that I added time as an eleventh category after realizing how the human body and its reactions change over time. The MI is interpreted as the combined score of all the individual categories' performance scores, similar to the way Olympic gymnastics athletes are scored as individuals and as a combined team. The MI is also similar in concept to the way university and college rankings, like the US News & World Report Best Colleges Ranking, tally an institution's overall score based on specific categories, like faculty research, entrance test scores, student retention, and alumni giving. Just as university rankings change each year, the MI varies with time as well.

To further define the categories for MI, I came up with numerous data elements for each category. For example, the sleep category comprises nine elements, the stress category thirty-three, and the food category approximately one hundred. The sleep category elements are hours of sleep, wake times, degree of dreaming, disturbances before sleep, physical sickness, environmental comfort, degree of overnight headache, degree of alertness in the morning, and degree of sleep-pattern disturbance.

By the time I'd fully defined each category, I had five-hundred elements that needed to be recorded and analyzed. It would be unrealistic, I realized, for anyone, including myself, to log hundreds of data points on a daily basis. Therefore, I designed the software so that, on a daily basis, a user would only have to manually input data for twenty-five elements. Data for the remaining elements data would be automatically generated through the computer, or artificial intelligence (AI). Developing the AI behind this technology involved figuring out the relationships among all eleven categories and subsequent five hundred elements. It has been one of my most difficult projects in my life. For instance, I applied seven years of self-study and four years of experience with psychotherapy to constructing the stress category, which ultimately took nine months to develop.

In summary, the MI comprises eleven categories, and within these eleven categories are five-hundred elements. A user only has to input data for twenty-five elements on a daily basis, so that's two to three element inputs per category. Based on the data entered, the app will automatically generate data for the other four-hundred and seventy-five elements. Once every element contains data, the app generates a score for each category. Once every category has a score, the app generates a total score, which is the user's MI value, or snapshot of their health condition. In simplified terms, the inter-connectivity among the categories (and the elements within them) is the mathematical model for human metabolism, and this mathematical model for human metabolism became the foundation for all my subsequent prediction models, including weight prediction, postprandial plasma glucose (PPG) prediction, and fasting plasma glucose (FPG) prediction.

While MI is a snapshot of overall health on any one day, the GHSU tells users about trends in their overall health. It's the three-month moving average of the MI, much as an A1C value is the average of your blood glucose levels over a three-month period. Using the MI and GHSU, I was able to determine my overall health state at any moment of any day.

Since developing the MI and GHSU three years ago, I've been logging all six input and all four output categories on a daily basis via the eclaireMD app (with the exception of lipid levels which cannot be checked every day). Each of these ten categories can be plotted out in graphic form over a selected time frame. For example, a user can view a line graph of their exercise and see that it is either increasing or decreasing over time. Below is an example of how I would enter data into eclaireMD.

MI and GHSU Categories

Input	Food	90% of past normal portion Carbs & sugar: 14 g per meal
	Exercise	18,000 steps (7.5 miles, or 12 km) per day
	Water	2,800 mL per day
	Sleep	Sleep: 7.2 hours per night
	Stress	99% score, or "almost no stress at all"
	Daily Routine Regularity	95% score
Output	Weight	170–175 lbs (BMI 25–26)
	Glucose	115 mg/dL
	Blood Pressure	105/64
	Lipids	LDL 99/HDL 45/Cholesterol 159/Triglyceride 115
	Total Score	**55–56 (Healthy)**

Healthy: 0–73.5   Unhealthy: 73.5+

This set of individual scores provides a combined score of 55–56 for my MI and GHSU, which means my health results are good and I am healthy. Physical examinations by my primary physician for the past three years have also confirmed my MI and GHSU health reports.

Originally, for the MI score, I had selected a random range of 0.5 (best condition) to 1.5 (worst condition). When both MI and GHSU are under 1.0, it means your health is generally good. If these values are over 1.0, you may have some health issues or related lifestyle problems. I chose an inverted scoring system, similar to golf and other medical health test scores, where a lower value score is better than a higher value score.

In most sports, the highest score wins. In my business career, increasing revenue numbers and raising profits quarter after quarter meant I was winning in the workplace. I had been born and raised in a developing country where scarcity was a way of life, but when I came to the US, I saw wealth and abundance everywhere. I was taught that bigger is better, more is great, and excess is a virtue. It's the American way. However, I believe this thought process and way of life is one of the reasons why Americans have become overweight and sick with chronic diseases. Excesses in food, drink, and stress, and a sedentary lifestyle, are overloading people's metabolisms and literally killing them.

Metabolic syndrome (which is a group of risk factors like high levels of blood sugar, blood pressure, lipid levels, and abdominal body fat) significantly increase a person's chances of developing heart disease and diabetes. Since MI measures the categories implicated in metabolic syndrome, I wanted an inverted scoring system that represented my ultimate goal, which was to lower my blood sugar, lower my blood pressure, lower my lipids, and lower my body weight. The only things I wanted to increase were water, sleep, and exercise (but only to optimal levels).

Eventually I decided to switch the MI scoring from a 0.5–1.5 range to a different inverted scoring system based on percentages. Using myself as a model, the "break-even" level for both MI and GHSU is 73.5 percent. Therefore, I consider any score above 73.5 percent as unhealthy and any score below 73.5 percent as healthy.

As of August 13, 2017, my MI and GHSU are at 56.6 percent and 55.2 percent, respectively, indicating that I am healthy. Over the past three years, my physicians have also confirmed, through various laboratory tests, that my general health is very good. I am an actual example of how one can control chronic diseases by applying quantitative methods to manage lifestyle scientifically.

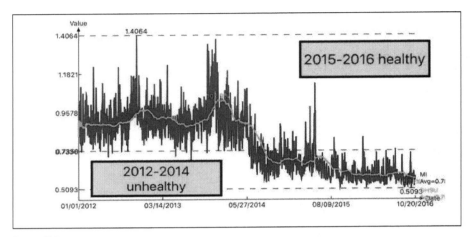

Figure 7-1:
MI & GHSU (2012–2016)

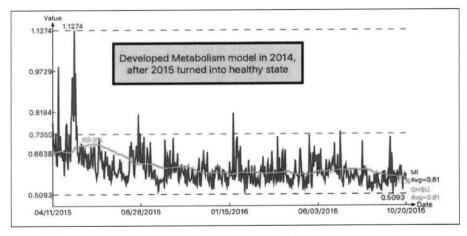

Figure 7-2:
MI & GHSU (4/11/2015–10/20/2016)

	A	B	C	D	E	F	G	H
1		Worst Condition	Best Condition	MI Score	MI Satisfaction Level (%)	Best Unit	Satisfaction Unit	
2	Water	1.5	0.7	0.74	95%	6	5.7	drink 5.7 bottles of water per day
3	Stress	1.5	0.5	0.51	99%			
4	Sleep	1.5	0.5	0.64	86%			
5	Sleep Hours	4	8	7.15	89%	8	7.15	sleep 7.15 hours per night
6	Wakeup Times	5	0	1.76	65%		1.76	wakeup 1.76 times per night
7	Food & Meal	1.5	0.5	0.73	77%			
8	Food & Meal Quantity	1.5	0.5	0.91	59%			
9	Food & Meal Quality	1.5	0.5	0.54	96%			
10	Daily Routine	1.5	0.7	0.74	95%			
11								
12								
13								
14								
15								
16								

Conversion table from individual category' score to satisfaction level. (5/11/2015 - 10/20/2016)

Figure 9-3:
Table Showing Conversion of MI Category Scores to Satisfaction Levels

A person's metabolism is the foundation of their overall health and, if managed poorly, the root cause of all chronic diseases. All the work I have done thus far on my medical project can be considered "preventive medicine" or "quantitative medicine"—medicine via physics and big data. I also call it "Save-Your-Own-Life Medicine!"

CHAPTER 8

YEAR FIVE
Weight and Post-Meal Glucose (2015)

Even before I was diagnosed with diabetes and a host of other health issues, I was aware of my increasing body weight, specifically in my mid-section. It was hard to ignore because I kept having to buy new pants, belts, and, eventually, suspenders to accommodate my growing belly. Looking back at old photos now, I can also see the weight gain in my face and neck. I remember having to buy new dress shirts with a larger neck size as well. Anyone who has ever gained weight over time can relate to the frustration of looking in the closet only to realize that nothing fits anymore.

Every time I moved up a shirt or pant size, it was like I was saying goodbye to the smaller person I once was and embracing my new reality as a heavier person. My weight gain never caused problems with my marriage, nor did it hinder my initial career ascent. Therefore, I wasn't motivated to reverse my situation. I simply thought of myself as the same person, only larger and heavier.

As I mentioned in Chapter 2, excess body fat, obesity, and inactivity are the highest risk factors for developing T2D. When I was officially diagnosed with T2D at the age of fifty, I was considered obese, at 220 pounds (99.8 kilograms). When I began my seven-year diabetes project at the age of sixty-three, I weighed 194 pounds (87.9 kilograms).

My increasing body weight was an indicator of many more negative health factors happening inside my body, including high blood pressure, high cholesterol, and high triglycerides.

Whereas I could only measure my cholesterol and triglyceride levels at blood testing facilities every few months, I could measure my weight, glucose, and blood pressure every day with tools I had at home, such as a weight scale, blood glucose monitor, and blood pressure arm cuff. Since lowering blood pressure is related to a healthy diet, increasing exercise, and lowering weight, I knew that to increase my health I should focus specifically on body weight and glucose. After spending all of Year Four (2014) developing a metabolism model (the foundation of my prediction tools in eclaireMD), I spent the following year developing a prediction tool for body weight and postprandial glucose (PPG), or post-meal glucose.

Weight Prediction

The reason I chose to develop my weight prediction software first was that body weight is one of the most obvious indicators of overall health. Most people learn to measure their own body weight before they learn to measure other general health indicators, such as cholesterol, blood pressure, and blood glucose. I'd venture to say more people own a weight scale at home than a blood pressure or glucose monitor. Also, an increase or decrease in body weight is more noticeable to the physical eye than fluctuations in internal health, such as cholesterol. Not only is body weight (and weight distribution) one of the most obvious signs of one's overall health, but it's one of the most important and easiest to monitor on a daily basis. Therefore, I chose to focus on developing a tool that could predict my weight in the morning (soon after waking and before breakfast).

I believe many people can relate to the feeling of stepping on a weight scale after returning from a weeklong vacation, or on the morning after a celebratory dinner, and thinking, "What's the damage?" Although it's normal for body weight to fluctuate as a result of events like vacations and holiday meals, weight gained over time becomes harder and harder to lose if we aren't vigilant about maintaining a healthy lifestyle. Also, what may work to reduce body weight in your twenties may not work as well in your forties or fifties because of decreasing metabolism. Therefore, the best way to practice preventive medicine is to maintain a healthy lifestyle based on your own metabolism model.

My vision was to be able to sit down at each meal and input the quality and quantity of food into my software program before I consumed the meal, and thus know what my weight would be the next morning if I consumed that meal. I could also input the quantity, type, and level of exercise performed that day and see how those factors would affect my weight the next day. Essentially, I wanted to find a way to quantitatively control the outcome of my weight the next morning through the decisions I made the previous day. Theoretically, using this prediction tool, I could go on a weeklong vacation and, without weighing myself each day, prevent unwanted weight gain.

Again using myself as the test subject, I measured and recorded the quantity of food I was consuming each day and my resulting body weight the next morning. I did this every day for three months and came up with a rudimentary weight prediction model. During this testing period I came to many conclusions. For example, I found that the quantity of food consumed was the most important influence on body weight. Food quality (processed versus natural foods), while a factor in overall health, did not affect resulting body weight as much as food quantity. Water intake was important, but I deemed it a secondary, or temporary, factor since water weight can be lost fairly easily via urination and sweat. Frequency of bowel movements was also a temporary factor, which could be influenced through consuming a high fiber diet.

The battle against weight gain is not a one-day effort. Eating less for one day doesn't guarantee weight loss the next day. Therefore, I used an accumulative three-day model. Over the subsequent three years, I measured and recorded my actual measured weight on a scale and compared it to the weight predicted by my software. I found that my weight prediction model had reached a 99.9 percent accuracy.

To calculate the accuracy of my daily predictions, my software would subtract my predicted weight from my recorded actual weight and then divide that difference by the actual weight value, which would produce a percentage known as the margin of error. The software would then subtract the margin of error from a perfect score of 100 percent. The resulting number would indicate the day's prediction accuracy percentage.

While it was important that each day's margin of error be as low as possible, what was more important to me was that the two numbers—predicted weight value and actual weight value—correlate with each other. For example, if my tool predicted I would gain weight the next day, then I wanted my actual weight to go up. Similarly, if I predicted I would lose weight the next day, then I wanted my actual weight to go down from the day before. When I plotted out my predicted weight values on a graph over the course of a month and overlaid that graph with my actual weight values over the same month, I saw two curves that moved together like twins. In statistics, this is called the "correlation coefficient" where two variables correlate with each other. Since the correlation coefficient of my predicted and actual weight was over 90 percent, I felt mathematically confident in my prediction model.

Post-Meal Glucose Prediction

About a month after I developed my weight prediction model, a conversation with my wife led to my development of a post-meal glucose prediction model. We were on our way to our favorite restaurant for breakfast, and I had been talking excitedly about how I came to finally develop my weight prediction model.

My wife, who often likes to look ahead to the next step, asked me, "Since your software can now predict weight, why don't you figure out a way to predict glucose after eating?"

I brushed off her question: "You don't know what you're talking about. Glucose is complicated because it's a nonlinear factor that is always changing over time. There are more variables that affect glucose than I can count. It's impossible!"

But the curious, scientific voice inside me kept asking, "Well, how many variables are there and how could I start measuring them?" I had used the word "impossible," which I typically don't like using because I had already accomplished so many things in my life that had been deemed impossible by others. Whenever the word "impossible" is thrown my way, my mind immediately starts trying to figure out how to make it possible. That's how my wife's question started me down the path to figuring out prediction of post-meal glucose. Clearly, she knows how to motivate me.

Within a month, I found a way. My first step was to list all the variables that could affect post-meal glucose. I came up with seventeen variables:

- amount of carbohydrates per meal
- amount of sugar per meal
- where the food is consumed (at home, restaurant, etc.)
- what type of food is consumed
- type of exercise
- length of exercise
- level of exercise
- amount of sleep
- quality of sleep
- stress level before the meal
- stress level after the meal
- time of glucose measurement (not beyond two hours after eating)
- time of day
- room temperature
- amount of medications
- type of medications
- time of medications taken

Once I'd developed my post-meal prediction model, I began comparing the predicted glucose values against my actual glucose values, which I measured through finger-prick blood tests three times a day every single day. Currently, I have more than three years' worth of data, totaling approximately 4,000 data points relating to post-meal glucose, including predicted and actual values. Using the same accuracy formula for my weight prediction model, the accuracy of my post-meal glucose prediction model is approximately 97 percent. The accuracy is not as high as the weight prediction model because of the numerous variables involved with glucose, but I believe it is high enough to deem the post-meal prediction model a success.

Being able to predict my post-meal glucose was a breakthrough for me, both scientifically and personally. On the scientific side, I proved glucose prediction could be done. On the personal side, figuring out how all the variables affected post-meal glucose meant I could manipulate those variables in my own life to lower my glucose without medication and improve my overall health.

Prior to developing the post-meal glucose prediction model, my daily exercise consisted of walking at least 10,000 steps a day, as measured with my pedometer. I would go about my normal daily activities, and if I had not met my quota by the end of the day, I would walk around my local park until I hit 10,000 steps. More often than not, the bulk of my daily steps were accomplished in the evening. I noticed that my post-meal glucose was usually lower after dinner than after breakfast or lunch, and I hypothesized it was because I was doing most of my exercise after dinner and before measuring my post-meal glucose. Therefore, I decided to break up my daily walking exercise of 10,000 steps into three major segments to be performed after breakfast, lunch, and dinner.

After finishing a meal, I would wait approximately thirty minutes to allow the food to digest a bit, and then I would start my walking exercise of 3,500–4,000 steps. I would plan to walk within two hours after each meal so that I could measure my post-meal glucose after the exercise was completed. After only a week of this new routine, I noticed exercise brought down my post-meal glucose values tremendously.

For example, I was on a low-carbohydrate diet, consuming only around 15 grams of carbohydrates at each meal. Combining three meals and snacks, I consumed a total of about 60 grams of carbohydrates per day. My data showed that one meal's 15 grams increased my post-meal glucose by thirty points. My data also showed that my exercise of 4,000 steps (equivalent to forty minutes of walking at 100 steps per minute, for a total of two miles, or three kilometers) decreased my post-meal glucose by twenty points. Therefore, the net glucose gain per meal with exercise was ten points, which meant I could maintain healthy glucose levels without medication.

By the end of 2015, I was thrilled to have lost enough weight to go from an extra-large to a medium shirt size, and from a 44-inch to a 38-inch waist pant size. Today, three years later, I am maintaining a 32- to 34-inch waistline. Furthermore, getting rid of my pot belly means I no longer need to wear suspenders!

As I mentioned earlier, up until the end of 2015, I had spent eighteen years taking three types of diabetes medication, including 2000 mg of metformin. Once I had lost weight and maintained healthy glucose levels with my prediction tools, I decided to gradually reduce all my diabetes medications—despite protests from my doctor. Within two years, I was able to stop taking my diabetes medications completely. Later, my physical exams would show that I was healthier off my medications than when I was on them.

After spending the last five years of my seven-year plan doing research and studying my own body, I came to the realization that the human body is a very powerful, sophisticated, and delicate system with tremendous capacity to repair itself. I believe God created this amazing system and we humans still don't understand it completely. I didn't want to disrupt my body's natural ability to heal itself by injecting unnecessary foreign agents into my body any longer. While there is a place for medication and surgery, I believe Western society has over-relied on these methods to treat many conditions, often making the conditions worse in the process.

During a routine physical exam in December 2015, my cardiologist, Dr. Jeffrey Guardino of Stanford Medical Center, and I discussed everything I had been doing for the past five years to control my diabetes. He was amazed at how much my overall health had improved. After I told him about my research and all the data I had collected on myself, he encouraged me to write a paper about it. At first, I scoffed at the idea. I was almost seventy years old and had never written a medical or health care paper before, nor did I have any desire to start doing so. That's when Dr. Guardino said to me: "Gerry, I have never seen a person who has over 1 million points of data about his own body, health, and medical conditions. Since the data is all within one host, you don't have to address different DNA or environmental influences. Your data can provide a lot of useful information to diabetes patients. More importantly, it can provide guidance to medical doctors." He planted a seed that day, but it would take almost another year for me to begin writing my first medical research paper.

CHAPTER 9
YEARS SIX AND SEVEN
Fasting Glucose (2016–2017)

I had now spent five years researching chronic diseases, developing the human metabolism model, and creating two major prediction tools for weight and post-meal glucose. The sixth year of research (2016) was relatively uneventful.

I had collected six to eight months' worth of health data on myself, but I needed more data over a longer period of time. Biomedical phenomena are dynamic and change over time. Therefore, the longer I collected consistent data, the more reliable my model and prediction tools would become.

So I continued to collect data and improve my software programs in the area of analytics. Although the software is meant to help users manage and improve their health, I also intended it to become a research tool that could collect and analyze both user data and AI-generated data. On a side note, I spent a great deal of time designing the input screens to reduce the chance of users inputting unnecessary or unrelated data (i.e., junk data). For example, the input design is very precise about what type of data can be input in each field, and very strict, so users must follow the input procedures exactly. This saves time and resources on data cleanup.

Having spent most of year six collecting and analyzing data, I realized I needed more of a challenge. I had remained physically active, walking at least four miles (six kilometers), or 8,000 steps, every day, but my mind needed to be just as active, if not more. In October 2016, I decided to take Dr. Guardino's advice and write my first medical paper; it would be a challenge, something I'd never done before. I did have experience writing mathematical research papers from my graduate school days, however. I approached my new task with the mindset of an engineer, attempting to avoid any personal prejudices and to present my methods, assumptions, findings, and conclusions in a straightforward and honest manner.

Up to this point, I had spent seven hours a day, 365 days per year, for six years, studying and researching diabetes. (Overall, I have dedicated approximately 18,000 hours to my seven-year project). When I first began writing, I didn't realize how much knowledge and information I had pent up inside of me waiting to pour out. Within two weeks, I had finished a first draft of one hundred pages. I titled it "Using Quantitative Medicine to Control Type 2 Diabetes." Over the next two months, I prepared and compiled almost seventy diagrams for the paper. Each diagram contained anywhere between one thousand to one hundred thousand data points that I had collected on myself for the past five years.

In the first draft of my paper, I used my A1C equivalent glucose (ninety-day averaged glucose) as my predicted fasting glucose. As a reminder, fasting glucose is one's blood sugar level after eight hours of fasting. It is typically measured in the morning after waking. I had found that my daily fasting glucose was always three to five points above or below my A1C. Since my fasting glucose had always been consistent in that regard, I assumed I could use my A1C as my predicted fasting glucose. A few years back, I'd met a doctor who had been treating diabetic patients for forty-plus years, and he told me that observing a patient's fasting glucose wasn't that important because it didn't change much. I had taken his assumption as medical fact and made the mistake of putting that assumption in my first draft.

I spent November tinkering with my diagrams. Toward the end of November, I flew to Hawaii to spend the fall and winter holidays with my family. As many people do around the holidays, I indulged a little more than normal during mealtimes, but still within healthful ranges. However, the day after Thanksgiving, my fasting glucose was 158 mg/mmol. This was a very unusual reading and I wanted to find out why. At first, I thought maybe my fasting glucose had been affected by the stress of traveling or being in a different environment. I had noticed before that I always tended to gain weight when

I was in Hawaii for an extended period of time, even if my physical activity and meal type and quantity remained the same. All I could do at this point was to continue to monitor my fasting glucose each day and see if it would go back to normal. After observing ten consecutive days of a higher-than-normal fasting glucose, ranging from 130 to 160, I went into a bit of a panic because I had no explanation for it. I had just completed my first medical research paper claiming that I was able to control my diabetes through quantitative medicine, and now my body was completely out of my control.

Back in California, my favorite place to take evening walks was at a local park. In Hawaii, my favorite place was in local grocery markets because of the air-conditioning. I don't care for the heat or humidity in Hawaii, so I try to avoid walking outdoors there. During my supermarket walks, I poured through the internet on my mobile devices searching for an answer to my fasting-glucose dilemma.

Every time I came across an article about how to affect fasting glucose, I would experiment on myself to see if the claims were true. For example, I came across one article that claimed the previous evening's post-meal glucose affected the following morning's fasting glucose, so I conducted a correlation analysis using my past post-meal and fasting glucose data and found no relationship between the two. Another article claimed that fasting glucose affected the morning's post-meal breakfast glucose, but after another correlation analysis, I found no relationship there as well. Yet another article recommended eating snacks or chewing candy before going to bed, which is horrible advice to anyone with diabetes or not. I tried that recommendation as well and it only made me gain weight and have bad breath in the morning.

I was so desperate to find answers that I even heeded one article's advice to wake up at 3 a.m. and measure my glucose every hour until daylight, so as to discover what type of high fasting glucose I had. This experiment not only degraded the quality of my sleep, but also threw off my glucose, weight, and metabolic index the next day. This activity was by far the worst one I tried and it didn't provide any more answers than I'd had when I started.

My daughter and her husband, who lived in Hawaii, suggested that perhaps the consistently warm and humid weather of the islands somehow was somehow affecting my fasting glucose. According to my research, while weather does not directly affect blood sugar, it can cause people to sweat more, move more or less, and eat different kinds of food, and those activities can affect blood sugar. To put the temperature theory to a quick test, I adjusted my room temperature during the night to see what kind of impact it had on my fasting glucose the next morning, but there was no significant relationship to be discovered.

I began year seven at a complete loss and didn't know what to believe or do next. By the end of January 2017, I had finished reading around 150 papers and articles on glucose, and I still had no clue how to answer my questions regarding fasting glucose. I wanted to know what causes it to increase, how high it can go, and, most important, how to control it. It was a big missing piece in my research paper.

By February, I was back in mainland U.S. continuing my search for answers. The hard-driving CEO, analytical engineer, and investigative scientist in me demanded answers. My fasting glucose continued to be high, averaging over 130 mg/dL, and I still couldn't find any mathematical trend or correlation to it. I thought about this dilemma so hard and often each day that I began dreaming about it at night. One night in mid-March, I woke suddenly at three in the morning from a dream, with an idea for finding answers to my questions.

All my training up to this point—in mathematics, computer science, physics, and engineering—was based on identifying inputs and outputs, developing equations, and then developing relationships between inputs and outputs to solve equations and predict outputs. Using these methods, I had exhausted all the statistical analyses between all the inputs, like food, sleep, and exercise, and the output of fasting glucose. However, in my dream, I had asked myself why I was looking at all the input categories, but not all the output categories. Could it be possible that one or more of the outputs was also an input that affects fasting glucose, a separate output?

Without meaning to, I had employed "out-of-the-box thinking," or taking a new or unconventional perspective on things. And it had come to me in a dream. After waking and going over my dream a few times to make sure I wouldn't forget it, I jumped out of bed and started to examine the correlation between output and output, as well as input and input. Four hours later, I had calculated that the correlation between my body weight and fasting glucose was as high as 80 percent. My "ah-ha" moment was discovering that my body weight had been the trouble maker this whole time!

I reviewed all my weight data from 2016 and saw that I had gone from 172 to 180 pounds (78 to 82 kilograms), a weight creep of about half a pound per month. Despite all my daily logging and use of my prediction tools, I hadn't been paying close attention to my overall weight gain. Upon further reflection, I realized I had begun gaining weight after one of my doctors advised me to eat more nuts to help lower my cholesterol. Nuts (e.g., pecans, cashews, macadamia, etc.) didn't affect my glucose, so I unconsciously ate too many of them each day. Certain nuts, including the ones I was eating, contain quite a bit of fat; they were the culprit in my steadily increasing weight. Since the weight gain had been so marginal each month, I had dismissed it as acceptable.

After realizing that the eight pounds (four kilograms) I'd gained had directly affected my fasting glucose, I began to quantitatively analyze how much my fasting glucose would increase by the amount of weight gained. On average, it increased about 20 mg/dL for every eight pounds of weight gain. Therefore, I was experiencing roughly a 3 mg/dL gain in fasting glucose for each pound of weight gained.

Using my knowledge of glucose and insulin production related to diabetes, I began to think about the biomedical link between weight and fasting glucose. I knew that the liver produces glucose for energy needs around three in the morning, and at the same time, the pancreas produces insulin to regulate the glucose. Since a diabetic's insulin does not work properly, the glucose is left unregulated and gets out of control in a diabetics' body.

I began to think about what controls internal organs like the liver and pancreas. That's when I thought about my father, who had passed away over twenty-five years earlier. He'd had a stroke that left him in a coma, and although he was declared brain-dead, his body continued functioning on life support. But, after two weeks, his body stopped functioning as well. The brain, I decided, must be the main controller of all internal organs, and if that was true, then the brain also had to give marching orders based on some kind of input. You can't have an output without an input. Going back to my engineering training, I asked myself, "What is the input that makes the brain tell the liver how much glucose to produce during fasting periods?" My hypothesis was that the answer was weight.

I had spent the last six years studying diabetes, not neuroscience, but I used my basic knowledge of system engineering to interpret this biomedical phenomenon and process. From an engineering standpoint, if I wanted my body to limit its outputs of X, Y, and Z, then I needed to control the inputs of A, B, and C.

I immediately began focusing on reducing my weight. However, I had an experience many people can relate to: my body resisted the effort to lose weight. The human body has evolved through thousands of years to prevent weight loss and promote weight gain by adjusting its metabolic rate. Fortunately, my personality is even more stubborn and persistent than my body, so I eventually got my body to give in and lose weight.

Because this book is not about how to lose weight, I won't go into specific detail about how I did it, but I will highlight one interesting discovery that helped me. I have many homes and travel quite a bit; therefore, I've established certain routines in each locale. As I mentioned before, I enjoy walking in a local parks in California and at large grocery markets in Hawaii. Although I can manage my diabetes and overall health anywhere, I've come to realize that certain environments encourage me to make better health decisions than others.

Back in late 2016, I had decided to purchase an apartment in downtown Vancouver, but I stayed there only from April to July of 2017. It was during this time that I lost the most significant amount of weight. Although environmental temperatures, as I mentioned previously, don't necessarily affect glucose directly, they may affect other behaviors that contribute to glucose and other output factors. For example, the heat and humidity of Hawaii meant I mainly exercised by walking in grocery stores, and grocery stores aren't that large; it can get monotonous walking in circles in such a tight space day after day. I likely walked the bare minimum. In Vancouver, however, the weather was perfect—just 60°F–68°F (16°C–20°C)—and my apartment was located near the Coal Harbor waterfront, where there was a long, beautiful walkway along the seawall with gorgeous views of the ocean and surrounding cityscape. Not only did I hit my walking quota each day, but I often exceeded it.

During my walks along the seawall and around Vancouver, I began to notice that most of the people I encountered were slim and healthy looking, regardless of their age, gender, or ethnicity. By comparison, I encountered numerous overweight people in California, Las Vegas, and Hawaii. I began to pay attention to other lifestyle factors in Vancouver, such as food portion sizes at restaurants, which were one-third to one-half less than in the United States. Also, many of the meals contained more vegetables and smaller portions of meat and bread. Another lifestyle factor was the amount of walking and biking Vancouverites were doing. While I was in Vancouver, the mayor got a new law passed to allow a separate bike lane on the bridge. The entire city appeared to be committed to a healthy lifestyle. Whenever I did observe overweight people there, I frequently discovered that they were tourists from the United States!

Being around so many people who practiced a healthy lifestyle was an eye-opener and affected me greatly. It motivated me to walk longer, walk more often, and eat even healthier. I didn't have a car, so I didn't drive anywhere, which greatly reduced my stress levels. Although I enjoyed being in California, my main complaint about the San Francisco Bay Area was the level of stress I felt from driving and being around so many people. In Vancouver, I felt no stress at all.

During my first two months in Vancouver, I didn't lose any weight, but I stubbornly continued to exercise and modify my diet until my body gave in. Within the next two months, my weight dropped quite consistently from 180 to 168 pounds (82 to 76 kilograms). Of course, I logged all this daily weight data, along with my fasting glucose, and plotted out the data on a graph. The lines in my weight graph and fasting-glucose graph were like a pair of twins, falling together from the top of the chart to the bottom.

During the month of July, I was doing one of my daily walks in a large, indoor shopping mall in the Richmond area when I came upon a store with a large tapestry on the wall that depicted the equation for Newton's Law of Gravity. I recalled how Newton came up with his theory of gravity after an apple fell from his mother's tree and hit him on the head. I suddenly felt I could relate to how he must have felt when that happened; discovering the relationship between weight and fasting glucose had been a similar lightbulb moment for me. Right there, under the tapestry depicting Newton's Law of Gravity, I pulled out my app and began reviewing my fasting glucose data from January 2014 to July 2017 and compared it with my weight data over the same time span and found they were most definitely linked: as weight declined so did fasting glucose. The relationship had been there the whole time, and I merely needed to discover it. Similarly, gravity had existed over millions of years waiting for Newton to make it known to the rest of the world. In all my research, I had read about how an increase in blood glucose could eventually lead to weight gain, but never about how weight loss could influence blood glucose.

By the end of July, I had developed a fasting-glucose prediction model that was very different from my post-meal glucose prediction model. It had taken me seven months of constant, daily effort (and nighttime dreaming) to finally figure out the solution to my problem. I was overjoyed, but I'm not the type of person to dwell on a success too long because I'm always looking for the next challenge to conquer.

EPILOGUE

Abu Dhabi, United Arab Emirates (December 2017)

I felt a swelling sensation in my chest as I crossed the finish line. Fortunately, although I was breathing a little heavier than normal, I wasn't having another cardiac episode. At the age of seventy, I had just completed my first 5K race, and the sensation I was feeling was sheer pride. As I looked around me, I saw numerous smiling faces and a shared sense of accomplishment. My daughter, who had completed the race with me, was also smiling, because she knew she didn't have to worry about my health anymore. I had come a long way from the days of late-night emergency transports to the hospital due to chest pains and other poor-health issues.

Eight months prior, I had not set out to participate in a 5K race. I had just completed my first research paper, the culmination of seven years of hard-won research and study. It was research I had performed on myself, resulting in over a million data points that proved I could save my own life without medication or surgery. Wanting to receive validation and feedback on my work, I submitted the paper to the International Diabetes Federation (IDF), the leading organization of the global diabetes community since 1950.

I chose the IDF because of its reputation, association with the United Nations, and official relations with the World Health Organization. I felt that if I was going to seek validation from any diabetes organization, it would be from the best and most well respected one in the world. Since I was new to the world of scientific research, publishing, and conferences, I wasn't entirely confident that my first-time effort at publishing research would be recognized by such a prestigious global organization. However,

I was entirely confident in what I had accomplished in the past seven years because I was living proof that my methods worked.

Two months after submitting my abstract (a 700-word summary of the paper), I received an email from the IDF stating that my paper had been accepted for poster display at their 2017 biennial conference in Abu Dhabi. Not only was I invited to present a 30-inch (76.2 cm) by 43-inch (108.4 cm) poster containing the highlights of my paper, but my abstract and poster would be included in their free and searchable online library as well. I was floored. Even though it had not been my main goal, it was hugely satisfying to receive outside validation for my years of hard work and painstaking data collection, research, and writing. Additionally, I was being given a platform to share my work and insights with the global diabetes community.

Although I had not originally set out, seven years ago, to write a research paper, nor to share my accomplishments on an international level, I somehow found myself on the cusp of doing just that. I was incredibly excited to dive into this new phase of my life and work. When I found out the conference was also hosting a 5K race for conference attendees, I immediately decided to sign up. I had never done anything like it before, but I was determined to embrace any new healthy lifestyle habits that were presented to me.

Having spent several years focusing on my own health issues, I found participating in a four-day international diabetes conference with 7,500 health care professionals from 182 countries to be an eye-opening experience. I arrived eager to share my research and methodology, and meet like-minded individuals from all over the world. To support me, my daughter also attended the conference so that she could network with other conference attendees on my behalf. Together, we could cover more ground, meeting with more individuals and making more connections.

Over a thousand posters were on display, mine among them, organized into categories. My poster was categorized under "Living With Diabetes— Diabetes Management," a category that contained only three or four other posters. I walked up and down the numerous poster display aisles, reading about topics that caught my eye and chatting up other poster authors. One author I met, a professor from Japan, was so impressed with my work that he invited me to his country to give a speech at a conference he was cohosting the following year. Another author was a medical doctor representing a governmental health and welfare organization in Bahrain. The conversation I had with him was one of the most interesting and encouraging. He was amazed by my prediction tool, and he, too, wanted to invite me to his country to speak about my research. All this positive feedback bolstered my confidence in what I had accomplished and was still accomplishing.

I had arrived at the conference focused on meeting other poster authors, but at my daughter's urging, I spent an afternoon speaking with delegates from diabetes associations representing individual nations. These were the public and government-sponsored diabetes associations charged with spreading awareness, educating consumers, and preventing diabetes. After speaking to these delegates, I found they all had one thing in common: Diabetes in all its forms, TD1, TD2, and gestational, was on the rise. These conversations enlightened me on the global diabetes epidemic, beyond U.S. borders.

I learned that in Ethiopia, basic awareness and education were a problem, as certain populations there believed holy water could cure them of the disease. I learned that in Cambodia, diabetes continues to affect younger and younger individuals as the youth consume more sugary drinks and processed foods than ever before. I learned that in Finland, TD1 is on the rise and no one knows why. I learned through the IDF itself that Asia is becoming the global epicenter for diabetes, with China and India leading the way, yet the countries are not doing enough to prevent and treat the disease.

Each country is on a diabetes-fighting spectrum, with the developing nations struggling with something as basic as access to proper health care and diabetes education, while developed nations have all the necessary awareness, education, and access to health care, but still have rising rates of the disease.

I've always believed that my prediction tool would benefit developing nations the most because it encourages diabetics to take charge of monitoring and maintaining their own health. This approach is essential in areas without regular access to health professionals or medical facilities. Also, because my prediction tool helped me to stop taking expensive medications for my diabetes and related chronic diseases, I hoped the tool would do the same thing for users in developing nations. Unfortunately, many at-risk populations in developing nations still don't have access to computers, mobile devices, or the internet. This is a hurdle I am still contemplating.

After one of the conference days, I decided to do some sightseeing at the Sheikh Zayed Grand Mosque. It was a beautiful sight to behold, the largest mosque in the country and, completed only ten years earlier, combining traditional and modern architecture. The building was covered in white marble, gold, semi-precious stones, and crystal. Its grand scale reminded me a bit of the Taj Mahal in India.

Before to the conference, I didn't know much about the United Arab Emirates (UAE) other than that it was a small, oil-rich country with the tallest building in the world. Looking around at all the modern infrastructure now, one would not suspect that a mere forty-six years ago, the country of UAE did not exist and the area contained a collection of tribes who mainly traded in pearls, fish, and livestock. In other words, before discovery of oil in the region and the founding president's foresight in investing oil money into building a modern future for the country, it had been a simple and quiet place.

Two things dawned on me. One, my own personal and professional rise in the United States mirrored the rise of UAE. Around the same time the UAE became a nation in 1972, I began my climb in American society. I invested in myself over and over again through education, self-study and learning, and starting businesses. Both the UAE and I have benefitted from investing in ourselves. The second thing I realized was that the Grand Mosque had been completed a decade ago, before I had started my seven-year plan.

My daughter reminded me that ten years ago to the day, we had traveled to India together. I had been unable to walk short distances without rest and barely able to climb stairs. We had taken a cycle rickshaw to reach the entrance to the Taj Mahal because I was worried I couldn't walk from the taxi drop-off to the entry gate. Now I was breezing through the thirty-acre Grand Mosque complex, and my daughter and I were signed up for the IDF 5K race later that evening.

It was my first 5K race, but I was confident that I could cross the finish line and barely break a sweat. I had predicted I would finish in approximately one hour and fifteen minutes, but the energetic feeling of the participants around me, combined with my daughter's faster pace, pushed me to finish in just under an hour. Surprisingly, I didn't notice much difference in my exertion level. This, I thought, is what it feels like to be healthy. Being healthy means you can focus on other things in your life because your body is working properly, instead of distracting or inhibiting you. Even though I had walked the entire race and was one of the oldest participants, I was not the last, not even near last, to finish!

Afterwards, my daughter and I took photos of ourselves at the finish line so that our friends and family could share our experience. The next morning, my daughter showed me side-by-side photos of myself—one taken in India in 2007 and one taken at the 5K finish line in 2017. The difference in my appearance was dramatic. In 2017, I had more gray hair, for sure, but the pot belly and the suspenders were gone. I was a "potato farmer" no longer!

This, my first diabetes conference, felt successful because I learned along the way and met some impressive individuals in the field. I could already tell this conference would be the launchpad for many other opportunities for me to share my work and, hopefully, help many others. As of this writing, I've completed twenty-two more papers based on my original data, and many of them were accepted by various other medical conferences and journals. I've also been invited as a keynote speaker to several of these conferences as well. Only time will tell where all this leads.

For so long, I'd considered being a successful CEO of a billion-dollar high-tech company to be the highlight of my career. I now consider the past seven years of study, research, and software development—all of which led to me restoring my health and saving my own life—as one of the true highlights of my life.

Working in high-tech, I believed I was helping others by making technology more efficient and useful, and providing greater access to information. Personally, I benefitted financially from being a high-tech CEO, but it nearly drove me into an early grave. I don't regret any part of my journey because it has brought me to the present day, where all my past experiences and knowledge have helped me to develop life-changing software prediction tools that can be held in the palm of your hand. For the next phase of my life, I truly hope to help people with what matters most, which is in their health.

I sold my company while I was at the top of my career because I came to realize that becoming professionally and financially successful should not come at the cost of one's life. At first, I struggled with the loss of my business. But I've come to appreciate how much I've gained since then. I have few responsibilities, and I have the financial freedom and time to pursue any and all interests I have, from breakthrough software development to nonprofit ventures. I also have more time to spend with family, and the wisdom and life experience to cherish it all.

I'm seventy years old, and I feel this is only the beginning.

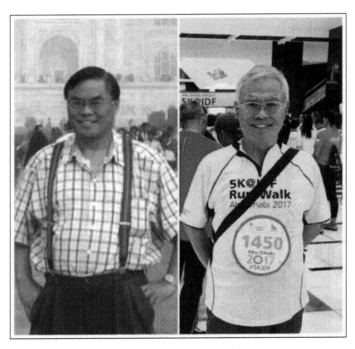

Before: December 2007 (Agra, India)
After: December 2017 (Abu Dhabi, UAE)

GERRY'S RULES FOR DIABETES MANAGEMENT

1. Maintain a healthy weight - Keep Body Mass Index (BMI) below 25.

2. If currently overweight, reduce daily food portions to 80% of normal amount.

3. Keep fasting glucose below 120 mg/dL by following the two rules above.

4. Keep carbohydrate/sugar intake below 15 grams per meal (a little less than the volume of one fist or one palm).

5. Eat fruit as a snack between meals, but not with meals.

6. Eliminate processed foods and drinks high in sugar, sodium, and unhealthy fats, usually found packaged in cans, boxes, and bags.

7. Walk at least twenty to forty minutes (2,000 to 4,000 steps) within two hours after every meal.

8. Keep postprandial (post-meal) glucose below 120 mg/dL by following rules 4 through 7.

9. Sleep at least six to seven hours per night, maintain a low-stress life, and drink 2,000 to 3,000 cc's (eight to twelve cups) of water each day.

10. Maintain regular physical check-ups and keep track of all health records.

Note: These rules are the author's personal guidelines that he follows. Always consult your physician before beginning any new diet or exercise program.

FINAL NOTE

Since the IDF conference in December 2017, I have written, presented, and published a total of 200 medical papers. I have attended more than fifty medical conferences and delivered approximately one-hundred speeches presenting my research. My GH-Method (math/physical medicine methodology) has been presented at more than twenty non-diabetes related conferences and I look forward to further contributing to the medical research field.

ACKNOWLEDGEMENTS

Foremost, I would like to express my deep appreciation to my former professors: Professor James Andrews at the University of Iowa, who helped develop my foundation in basic engineering and computer science, and Professor Norman Jones at the Massachusetts Institute of Technology, who taught me how to solve tough scientific problems through the right attitude and methodology.

I wish to express my appreciation to my son-in-law, Duff Janus, who suggested I write this medical memoir; and my daughter, Cindy Janus, who helped bring my voice and story to life within these pages.

I also wish to thank my son, John Hsu, who continues to inspire and contribute to my diabetes research.

I owe a deep debt of gratitude to my father for passing along his wisdom to me and exposing me to the medical world; and to my mother for raising me to be persistent and to have strong will power in life.

Last, but not the least, I'd like to acknowledge and thank my beloved wife, Li Li, who is the best partner anyone could have. Her tireless love, encouragement, and support for everything I've done in my life has made all the difference.

REFERENCES

Centers for Disease Control and Prevention. (2014). *Diabetes home.* Retrieved from: https://www.cdc.gov/diabetes/data/statistics/2014statisticsreport.html

Diabetes Canada. (2017). *Diabetes statistics in Canada.* Retrieved from: http://www.diabetes.ca/how-you-can-help/advocate/why-federal-leadership-is-essential/diabetes-statistics-in-canada

National Institute of Diabetes and Digestive and Kidney Diseases. (2016). *Diabetic kidney disease.* Retrieved from: https://www.niddk.nih.gov/health-information/diabetes/overview/preventing-problems/diabetic-kidney-disease

U.S. Department of Health and Human Services Office of Minority Health. (2016). *Diabetes.* Retrieved from: https://minorityhealth.hhs.gov/omh/content.aspx?ID=6780

U.S. News & World Report. (2017). *Best medical schools: Research.* Retrieved from: https://www.usnews.com/best-graduate-schools/top-medical-schools/research-rankings

United States Census Bureau. (2016). *Monthly & annual retail trade.* Retrieved from: https://www.census.gov/retail/index.html?eml=gd&utm_medium=email&utm_source=govdelivery

United States Department of Agriculture Economic Research Service. (2017). *Food consumption & demand.* Retrieved from: https://www.ers.usda.gov/topics/food-choices-health/food-consumption-demand/food-away-from-home.aspx

World Health Organization. (2017). *Diabetes.* Retrieved from: http://www.who.int/diabetes/en/

Yale School of Medicine. (2010). *Endocrinology & metabolism.* Retrieved from: http://endocrinology.yale.edu/news/article.aspx?id=1366

Made in the USA
Lexington, KY
10 November 2019